Yoga

Master Yoga Poses While Strengthening Your
Body, Calming Your Mind and Be Stress Free

(Yoga Philosophy for Mindfulness, Yoga Lifestyle
and Happiness)

Julia Solloway

Published by Rob Miles

Julia Solloway

All Rights Reserved

ISBN 978-1-989990-60-5

Legal & Disclaimer

The information contained in this book is not designed to replace or take the place of any form of medicine or professional medical advice. The information in this book has been provided for educational and entertainment purposes only.

The information contained in this book has been compiled from sources deemed reliable, and it is accurate to the best of the Author's knowledge; however, the Author cannot guarantee its accuracy and validity and cannot be held liable for any errors or omissions. Changes are periodically made to this book. You must consult your doctor or get professional medical advice before using any of the suggested remedies, techniques, or information in this book.

Table of Contents

INTRODUCTION

Most people experience back pain from time to time. A lot of people have looked for cure, but does not work, or was really suitable for them, so Whether this pain is severe and chronic or mild and short-lived, the most of time, it causes misery and curtails everyday activities. Why we do not listen to our bodies and minds this is a metaphorical expression, but what I mean is why we do not practice yoga for back pain? Yoga has been associated with healing through the millennia. It is without cost, self-administered, and silent, and it demands no equipment beyond a pillow, a belt, or a chair. Yoga relieves pain and promotes calm to endure any pain that remains. It can address back pain generally, through prevention, and directly with attention to the specific cause of existing pain. No special beliefs are required in the practice of yoga. This a book provides with everything you need about Yoga, explains the causes that lead to back pain; how to deal with them, it offers you the major basics of the upper, and low back. It offers you the major instructions and poses that will empower your mind and body with practicing Yoga with simple tools.

Therefore, Yoga means "yoke" (a link, a harness that joins together) or "unity." This unity refers to the oneness of body and mind. The purpose of yoga is to bring together the body and mind to create harmony or well-being. The word yoga also means "discipline" or "effort."

Some people think of yoga as an art; others call it a science. Most would agree that although it is associated with Hinduism, it is a secular practice that can be done by individuals of any faith or no faith. I like to think of yoga as a system of behavior that encompasses mankind's social context; that is, it exists in a social environment, influencing and being influenced by the community around it.

Certainly, yoga has gathered devoted practitioners from many different faiths and lands. The classical form of yoga has eight limbs, or branches, the first two of which are relevant for anyone who considers using yoga to aid in the healing process, to relieve back pain or any other type of pain.

So, whether you are beginner or advancer this does not matter with this a guide you will learn and teach yourself with this a book, by following the instructions and pictures which have been included. This a book covers the Backgrounds about Yoga and Back Pain, The major features of Yoga for Back Pain, The Techniques and Styles of Yoga, The Major Features of Back Pain and last chapter The Instructions and Poses of Yoga for Back Pain.

In this a book which under title **How to Use Yoga Poses for Back Pain,** in which you will find out plenty information and ideas not only about back Pain which a center idea, but you will also discover other interesting features such as breathing exercises (....), it also provides with philosophical versions and the best methods in Yoga, in which anyone should practice Yoga in everywhere they are and exist, even at their work, at home and at garden with simple tools.

Chapter 1: Yoga: An In-Depth

Understanding

As Yogi Bhagavad Gita said in one of his teachings, "Yoga is the journey of the self, through the self, to the self."

Generally, most of us are accustomed to seeking fulfillment from things and people in our immediate surroundings and hardly perceive fulfillment as an inner feeling. Nevertheless, different experiences we go through help us understand that no external factor has the potential to fulfill our deep longing for satisfaction and fulfilment. Unfortunately, most of us often gravitatetowards action instead of awareness. In this state, we lack awareness of our surroundings, the present, and ourselves which is why we are never fully content with our lives or ourselves.

As a practice, Yoga helps you achieve a state of total calmness, tranquility, and contentment. Yoga is the ultimate answer to the longing, yearning, and chaos we feel inside, and outside us. So, what exactly is yoga?

Yoga is a practice that reverses the routine outward energy flow and consciousness, making your mind the dynamic hub of perception; allowing it to stop reliance on your fallible senses, and become capable of properly experiencing the truth.

Yoga is a mental, spiritual, and physical discipline that originated sometime in the fifth and sixth centuries BCE in India. The term 'yoga' comes from the word 'yuj', a Sanskrit word meaning 'to bind' or 'to yoke'. A common interpretation of yoga is as discipline or union. Male and female yoga practitioners bear the names 'yogi' and 'yogini', respectively.

Yoga unites your body, mind, and soul by making use of the eight yoga sutras; sutras are the eight elements in your body that can help you attain enlightenment.

Yoga Sutras

Yoga sutras, also referred to as the eight-limbed path or eight-fold path are as follows:

1. The Yamas

The first sutra is the 'Yamas' which are the behavior patterns or ethical standards describing how you need to live your life. The Yamas include 'ahimsa' which means practicing non-violence and not harming anyone, 'Satya' which means being truthful, 'Asteya' which translates to not stealing anything from anyone, 'bramacharya' which refers to exercising self-restraint, and 'aparigraha' which refers to non-covetousness.

2. The Niyamas

Niyamas are the second Sutra, and refer to developing an attitude of self-discipline. The Niyamas set guidelines for healthy, clean, and good living. They include 'Saucha' which means cleanliness, 'Samtosha' which refers to contentment and being modest, 'tapas' meaning cleansing your body of impurities and staying healthy, 'svadhyaya' which translates to 'self-inquiry' and lastly, 'isvara pranidhana' meaning surrendering to your God.

3. Asanas

The third factor is 'Asanas' which are the physical positions practiced in yoga. Your body serves as a temple for your spirit, which is why it is your duty to care of it, and ensure it always remains healthy and in a fit state. By practicing various Asanas, you can purify and detoxify your body, and enhance your ability to properly focus, meditate, and concentrate.

4. Pranayama

Pranayama is the fourth sutra, which means controlling your breathing. By regulating your breathing movements with the help of breathing exercises, you make the best use of'prana', the energy living inside you. By doing so, it rejuvenates your body, and increases your average lifespan.

5. Pratyahara

Pratyahara is the fifth sutra; it means directing your attention inward. Practicing Pratyahara helps yourealistically understand yourself through observing your habits, cravings, and desires, and is thus able to eliminate all negative traits from your personality.

6. Dharana

Dharana, the sixth sutra, refers to concentrating on your mind with proper focus and energy. By concentrating on one thing in particular, it helps augment your focus and the ability to be attentive on just one thing at a time.

7. Dhyana

The seventh sutra, dhyana, refers to contemplation or meditation. Meditation helps you attain stillness and calmness, which gives you further and better insight into your mind.

8. Samadhi

Samadhi is the eighth sutra and refers to a state characterized by continual ecstasy or bliss. This state commonly refers to as state of enlightenment, where you make good use of all the seven sutras mentioned above, and are able to derive the benefits they offer to acquire nirvana. If you devote to the regular practice of yoga, strive to achieve perfection in it and explore it deeper, you will be able to objectify the state of nirvana.

Yoga As A Way Of Life

Contrary to popular belief, yoga is deficient of strong religious ties. Yoga is a way of life that helps you improve your quality of life, and acquire peacefulness in every aspect of life. People belonging to different religions across the globe practice yoga to deepen their spiritual and religious beliefs, and achieve a state of complete awareness and serenity.

Physical yoga commonly practiced worldwide is hatha yoga. Hatha yoga is a combination of sun and moon postures. Sun postures are heating postures (postures that heat up your body), while moon postures are postures that cool down your body. By using hatha yoga, you energize, as well as calm down your body.

This guide is going to shed some light on different hatha yoga postures and practices. By engaging in, and practicing these poses, you will enjoy the following benefits:

Stress, Anxiety, and Depression Relief: Yoga helps you connect to the portions of your brain responsible for regulating stress; by tapping into these areas of your brain and exercising them, you gain complete freedom from stress, anxiety, and depression.

Lose Weight: Yoga energizes your body and enhances your metabolism. When your metabolic rate enhances, you burn calories at a faster pace, a fastened heart rate is a critical factor in healthy weight.

Become Happier: By eliminating stress from your life and body, you become calmer which improves your emotional well-being, making you feel happier. Moreover, different yoga poses improve serotonin levels in your body (serotonin is a mood-boosting hormone). This enhances your state of happiness.

Improve Your Health: Various yoga poses reduce inflammation in the body, stabilize your blood cholesterol and sugar levels, detoxify your body, regulate your blood pressure, and keep your heart healthy. All these factors improve your immune system and health, keeping various serious bodily ailments and disorders at bay.

Focus Better: By practicing yoga postures aimed at enhancing your concentration, you can improve your focus and attention span. This helps you efficiently manage your time and increase productivity.

Become More Creative: By using various yoga poses designed to improve your thinking and creative abilities, you can improve your innovative skills and become better at coming up with unique ideas.

Builds Strength, Muscles, and Protects Your Bones: By performing different yoga poses aimed at enhancing your physical and muscular strength, you build more muscle mass, and strengthen your bone; this reduces bone loss, tissue inflammation, and keeps you safe from conditions such as arthritis.

Yoga Improves Your Body Posture: Most physical problems stem from having a bad posture. Yoga can easily correct this problem. All yoga poses help improve your body posture and when you correct your posture, your physical health improves.

Yoga Combats Insomnia and Sleep Related Problems: In addition to the aforementioned benefits, by reducing stress, improving your well-being, and enhancing your calmness, yoga cures insomnia and treats various sleep related problems.

Yoga Increases Self-Esteem and Confidence: Yoga helps you understand yourself better, gives you peace of mind, and gets rid of negative, poisonous thoughts that lower your self-worth and confidence. When these changes take place in your body, your self-esteem, and confidence start perking up.

Yoga Improves Your Awareness: Yoga gives you a chance to be cognizant of the present and value it. Moreover, it improves your awareness and mindfulness, which helps you live a better life.

To enjoy these benefits, start practicing yoga today! In the next few sections, we shall outline different yoga poses you can practice to improve your quality of life.

CHAPTER 2: YIN & YANG

In the last chapter, I mentioned that Yin Yoga is entirely different from the Yang practices. But how is it different? While there are differences in the postures, their names, and how we hold them, what exactly is the differentiating factor? Unless we get a clear idea of what Yin and Yang are, our yoga practice is bound to remain incomplete.

Yang is dominant while Yin prefers to remain dormant. In other words, Yin and Yang are antonym patterns that we see and experience daily. They are two sides of the same coin. When they are in sync and balance, life is peaceful and healthy. The slightest disharmony could also shed a deep darkness in any or all aspects of our lives.

Like the two sides of the coin, Yin and Yang co-exist. They are dependently independent. Since our lives are never static, these two are always in the flow, constantly changing.

Each and every living being on this earth display the Yin and Yang attributes. Like the shade which is dependent on the existence of light, Yang depends on how strong the Yin is. You can compare them in numerous ways. If Yang is masculine, Yin is feminine. Yang is active; Yin is gentle. Yang is superficial, but Yin lies deep within us. Yang is evident; Yin is mysterious.

If Yang is hot, Yin is cool. Yang is the Sun and Yin, the moon... The comparisons seem to be endless, but all of them just point out to only one concept. Nothing in this world is complete without these two contrasting elements in a certain pre-designed proportion.

Since the Yang is active and dynamic, the global Yoga flows which we practice [Hatha, Ashtanga, Power and others] can be considered as Yang. On the other hand, in the Yin, we tend to follow our breath in a passive way.

17

The Yin-Yang Connection

Yin transforms into Yang, but this transformation could be slow and steady or sudden, depending on the trigger. As we move into the day from a sleepy night, the Yin fluidly moves into Yang. The same is applicable as winter paves the way for spring. On the other hand, when summer moves into fall, we slow down, allowing Yin to become dominant.

At times our energies undergo a sudden transformation. If we are caught up amidst some physical or emotional hurricane, we can experience this turbulent change. However, if our energies are balanced, then the change stabilizes soon.

It might look as if the dominant Yang is the controller. But, alas! The Yin, the feminine energy that is subtle and silent, controls the masculine energy. When the Yang starts increasing in an uncontrollable way, it throws our lives out of balance. The universe then steps in to restore the natural balance in some form or other.

In the same way, an excess of Yin energy is also not acceptable as it could put us under tremendous fatigue (physically, emotionally, spiritually), eroding away the balance.

And, this is why respected teachers across the world emphasize on striking a balance. Our lifestyles, these days, are quite far from this balance. We are always under stress, triggering the Yang energy. In the process, we tend to suffer from numerous health conditions. Depression, stress, anxiety attacks, obesity, chronic digestive disorders – these are some of the most widely seen ill-effects of Yin-Yang imbalance.

While active yoga practices do wonders in offering relief to all the states mentioned above, the deep-seated tissues often succumb to these perils. And, that is why we need to practice Yin Yoga as well. Being restorative in nature, this style offers you a chance to balance your uprising Yang. It gives an opportunity to eliminate the piled up energy in a calm way.

Since they are not separate from each other, through a dedicated and particular practice, we'll able to harmonize and balance their energies, ensuring a happier, healthier life.

Chapter 3: Cow Pose / Bitilasana

One of the beginner poses, Cow Pose is easy to perform. The pose is named thus as bitila in Bitilasana, the Sanskrit name for the pose, means"cow". It is generally paired with Cat Pose. The pose, though simple, offers amazing health benefits.

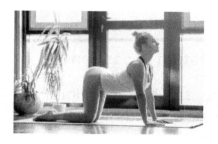

How To Do Cow Pose

Go on fours by placing your hands and knees on the floor. Your hands should be in line with your shoulders and knees should be aligned to your hips. Ensure hip-width distance between your knees. You will now resemble a tabletop.

Let your head be neutral with the gaze fixed on the floor.

With inhalation, lift your buttocks up towards the ceiling as your chest goes slightly inward.

Gently push your belly downwards while drawing your chest upward. Expand your shoulders. At this stage of the pose, your spine will be curved downwards.

Lift your head to look straight.

Exhale and return to position.

Repeat the steps 10-20 times or for 1 minute, as slowly as desired.

Don't forget to breathe and try to exhale when releasing.

As mentioned above, Cow Pose is often integrated with Cat Pose and hence when performed together they make a sequence. This creates the ultimate benefits. We will dive into Cat Pose, next, in Chapter 3.

Benefits of Cow Pose

The benefits of Cow Pose include:

Stretches the neck and spine

Tones back muscles

Improves posture

Stretches the front part of the body

Increases lung capacity

Stimulates abdominal organs for optimum functioning

Relieves back pain

Reduces sciatic pain

Supports pregnancy phase and prepares for labor

Improves balance

Relieves anxiety and promotes calm

Note

Those with neck pain can perform the pose without lifting the head. In case of chronic neck condition or neck injury, it is best to refrain from practicing the pose.

Using Props

If your knee hurts as you go on fours, you can place a blanket under your knees to relieve the pain and focus on performing the pose.

CHAPTER 4: LIMBERING UP

Before you can reach those subtle sensations that are mentioned in the quotation above, you need to understand that your body, as a beginner to yoga, is not accustomed to the exercise you are about to give it. Therefore, you need to limber up and get each part of the body ready for the exercises which follow.

Limbering up is a simple task and once you become accustomed to it, you will find it will become a part of your yoga practice. The purpose that it serves is that it prepares your body for exercise and makes you much more conscious of your body's need to break into these exercises gently. The warming up or limbering up process before you begin your exercise routine is vital. It helps your circulation,

Exercise 1 – Limbering up – Feet and hands

The first exercise will help you to prepare your wrists and your feet to be more flexible and ready to exercise. You will not be expected to twist your feet into the Lotus position until later because this isn't a beginner exercise. Thus, don't be put off by images of having to be that flexible. To limber up, hold your arms out in front of you and relax the hand and wrist. Make it totally limp and then shake your hand up and down. Then shake it side to side. Repeat the process for the other arm. You may find as you advance that you can do both at once, but be totally aware of the limb that you are working on.

If you watch athletics, you will notice that sportsmen and women always limber up before performing. This is for a very good reason. They are preparing their bodies for the exercise which is to come and in yoga, you are doing the same thing, but you are becoming more and more aware of your body.

Now hold your foot out in front of you. Relax the foot. Be aware that your foot is relaxed and then wobble the foot, so that you feel the muscles around your ankle become more flexible. You can also use a rotation of your foot after you have practiced simply wobbling the foot, but at the beginning stages, just imagine your foot as totally relaxed.

Exercise 2 — Limbering up — Neck and shoulders

For this area of the body, you need to be totally aware of the strains and stresses which life has imposed upon you. These generally center on the spine and the neck and shoulders take the most strain because the energy flows to that area when you tighten up and tense the body. Thus, before you start to perform head rolls or shoulder rolls, you need to warm this area up with limbering up exercises. Breathe in and breathe out as you did when you were lying down. You can do these limbering up exercises seated or standing, but you do need to be aware of the feelings that your body emits. Such feelings may be that your neck or shoulders are tense or that they are relaxed. Learn to listen to your body as you limber up. As you breathe in and out, concentrate on your shoulders and allow them to relax, lift them up slightly, and then relax them. Don't try anything more energetic than simply being aware of your shoulders and wiggle them around a little so that your awareness increases. Then relax. Repeat this several times to give your shoulders the preparation that they need.

Exercise 3 – Limbering up – Elbow touching

This is a particularly good exercise for limbering up the shoulder area. Place your fingertips onto your shoulders. Keeping them there, lift your arms to shoulder height and move your arms forward until they touch. Breathe normally during this process. Move the arms back and relax. Repeat this three to four times.

For the neck area, be aware of where you suffer stiffness. Wobble your head from left to right. The idea of the warming up exercises is to simply relax each part of the body and move it so that you know your own weaknesses and strengths. It's not about vigorous exercise at this stage or about hurting yourself. It's about being aware and preparing your body for the exercises which follow in later chapters. Young people may think that they can just jump into exercises, but the limbering up exercises are vital to beginners who have the impression that exercise means exertion. It's about familiarizing yourself with your body's needs and being aware of who you are and what you feel.

Exercise 4 – Limbering up – Waist and body area

As you have wobbled different areas, you may be a little curious as to how you can wobble your waist. In the limbering up stages, you can actually make this fun. Imagine that you have a hula hoop and rotate your body as if keeping this in place. If you actually have one, use it because, at any age, this helps you to limber up the center area of your body.

CHAPTER 5: YOGA FOR BEGINNERS:

UNDERSTANDING YOGA

We live in a stressful busy world. With so many things demanding our attention, it is very easy for stress, anxiety and depression to be a norm in our life. Ultimately, this could easily make us to live very unhappy lives even when everything seems to be perfect in the eyes of outsiders. Our minds seem to be constantly thinking about stuff that has nothing to do with our present moments. We are so engrossed in thoughts about the past (regrets, blames etc.) and the future (worries, anxieties etc.) that we barely notice the beauty of the moments that we have every minute. When you couple that with our changing ways of life such as living a sedentary life, the result has been an unhealthy generation that is wallowing in stress, anxiety and depression. While different physical exercises do help to alleviate stress, anxiety and depression, the truth is that they do have their own limitations. For instance, you can engage in physical activity while your mind is far away in a distant future or past. Even if you might derive some benefits that come with the physical activity e.g. improved fitness, the truth is that you could do a lot better if you could ground your thoughts to the present so that you can enjoy moments as they unravel as opposed to thinking about the future or the past unnecessarily. That's what makes yoga a perfect solution to many of the problems associated with mindlessness (being obsessed about the future or the past) and sedentary living. Why is that so? Well, because yoga is more of a blend between mindfulness meditation (you practice this through breathing techniques and other forms of mindfulness meditation) and specialized physical activity (asanas), which could ultimately help you to derive benefits you perhaps never thought possible. Yoga goes further than any physical activity can as far as ensuring that you derive the benefits of physical activity in that it can help target some parts of your body that would be very difficult to target while engaging in other physical activities.

So what exactly is yoga?

The term 'yoga' is derived from the Sanskrit word 'yuj', which when loosely translated means union. In this case, yoga means the union of universal consciousness with individual consciousness/soul. That can only happen when you are mindful of every moment as it arises. The thing is; yoga is not just the physical movements i.e. asanas, which entail twisting, turning, stretching and breathing; it also aims at unleashing the infinite potentials of the human mind and soul through meditation. In other words, yoga, as described by Sri Sri Ravi Shankar, is not just exercise coupled with asanas (the yoga poses are referred to as asanas) but the emotional integration along with spiritual elevation that have a touch of mystic element that have the potential of giving you an understanding of something beyond your imagination.

Dating back to as early as over 10,000 years ago, yoga has evolved from what it was originally meant for (mainly for helping yogis to unleash their spiritual and mental potential) to everyday use where it is no longer a preserve of any religion. Today, yoga has become a global practice with more people engaging in it for purposes other than spiritually inspired aims.

Yoga's increasing popularity as a physical/mental exercise among people of all ages, cultures, and religions links back to its ability to help combat stress, depression, and anxiety in a world and age that has taken over by constant stress and unending race to stay ahead of industrial, business, and academic competitions.

What makes yoga such a powerful exercise for taking care of mental and physical conditions? Let us look at some scientific explanations to yoga's effectiveness.

The Science Behind Yoga

High stress, anxiety and depression levels increase the production of cortisol, a major stress hormone. Cortisol keeps you alert during crisis. However, prolonged secretion can disturb your body's functioning resulting to a wide array of health complications.

When you engage in yoga, it lowers your stress levels, which leads to the reduction of the amount of cortisol secreted into the body and increased level of relaxation and calmness.

Yoga's ability to reduce the production of Cortisol also explains why yoga helps strengthen your immunity. Why is that so? Well, excessive production of Cortisol can reduce the strength of your immune system by immobilizing your defense system. Reducing Cortisol production through yoga ensures this does not happen.

Further, studies have shown that engaging in yoga helps stimulate the parasympathetic nervous system. The stimulation of the parasympathetic nervous system boosts the flow of blood to the digestive organs, endocrine glands, and all other vital organs in your body, thereby reducing your heart rate, anxiety levels, and blood pressure, thus helping you live a happier life.

With that understanding, let's take the discussion a bit further where we will discuss the benefits that come with practicing yoga.

Benefits of Practicing Yoga

Yoga has several benefits most of which focus on health and health-related issues. Let us look at some of yoga's most notable benefits as well as what makes yoga such an effective way to derive these health benefits.

Boosts Immunity

According to one Norwegian study, engaging in yoga can lead to significant changes in the gene expression responsible for boosting immunity at the cellular levels. These changes do not take long to occur as they can happen while you are still lying on your yoga mat.

Mitchel Bleier, a researcher who runs a yoga studio in Connecticut, believes that yoga's ability to boost your immunity links back to the fact that yoga helps improve your breathing, movement, and circulation. Improved breathing, movement, and blood circulation leads to the optimal functioning of every vital organ in your body. This ultimately leads to a boost in your level of immunity.

The Sun Salutation is one of the many yoga poses that can boost your immunity.

Helps Reduce Migraines

According to research, people who experience constant migraines suffer less migraine-related pains after engaging in yoga exercises for a period of 3 months. While there is no proof to what really causes migraine, researchers such as Mitchel Bleier believe migraine develop from a combination of physical misalignment and mental stressors that on top of causing migraine, also cause several other health problems.

Stressors and physical misalignments such as hunching over a cell phone or PC with your head stretched forward and shoulders up could lead to the excessive lifting of your trapezius and cause a tightening around your neck. This can pull your head forward and create an imbalance in your neck muscles leading to migraines and headaches.

Yoga poses that involve lifting the back of your chest towards the chin and drawing the chin away from the chest are ideal for bringing you this yoga benefit. One example of such yoga poses is the bridge pose that can make the upper trapezius muscles to effortlessly flow away from your head.

Ideal for Boosting Your Sexual Performance

Studies by Bleier and his team have shown that engaging in yoga asanas for 3 months can boost libido, sexual arousal, orgasm, confidence, and sexual satisfaction in men and women. This is because yoga poses improve blood circulation and the flow of blood into the genitals; this increased blood flow is vital for healthy arousal and performance during sex.

Further, your ability to control your mind and breathe during yoga can also improve your performance and concentration during sex. The ability of yoga exercises to strengthen the floor muscles also helps improve sexual performances.

Yoga poses that bring your knees closer to the ground, move your groin back, and engage the pelvic floor muscles are great for achieving this end. The bound angle pose comes in handy here thanks to its ability to open the hips and engage the pelvic floor muscles to improve orgasm.

Improved Sleep

Harvard researchers have proof that engaging in yoga exercises daily for 2 months greatly improved the quality of sleep enjoyed by insomnia patients. Another study by Bleier and his team also suggests that engaging in yoga at least two times per week can also help cancer survivors get better sleep at night. This is because of yoga's ability to deal with stress and anxiety more effectively.

Stress and anxiety make your head run in circles and relaxing becomes next to impossible. On the other hand, engaging in yoga can help you breathe deeply, relax your jumbled nerves, slow your heart rate, and enjoy peaceful sleep.

Poses that call for lying on your back as you practice deep breathing, poses such as the corpse pose, are ideal for improving your sleep.

Helps Combat Excessive Food Cravings

According to Washington University researchers, engaging in regular yoga practices can link back to an increased awareness of all emotional and physical sensations that go along with eating. The breath awareness that goes with yoga helps improve the connection between your mind and your body.

Yoga helps you become more attuned to the emotions that go along with cravings for certain foods; this attunement helps you slow down and make wise choices whenever these food cravings hit you. Coupling deep breathing meditation with any sitting yoga pose can help you control your food cravings.

Deep breathing is at the core of every yoga practice. Let us look at how the breath affects the body and how you can harness the benefits of deep breathing as you practice yoga.

Chapter 6: Deep Rhythmic Breathing

Man derives more energy from the air he breathes than from any other single source. While the human body can subsist for several weeks without food, it cannot live deprived of air for even a short time. The yogis call oxygen 'prana'. Man absorbs prana from the air through breathing. Prana is present as a vital force in everything; it is in the food you eat and the water you drink. The yogis believed that there exists an unexplainable relationship between prana and the mind, and this is why they stressed the importance of proper breathing. Rhythmic breathing exercises were combined with physical postures of the body because the yogis found each worked to greater advantage when done with the other.

Fresh air and correct breathing habits are among the most valuable privileges of humanity, yet most people have little conception of their importance and proper use. We do shallow breathing of from the chest, absorbing only a limited amount of oxygen. Through special deep rhythmic breathing, the amount of oxygen that we take in can be greatly increased.

Breathing is the most essential biological function of the body. Civilized man has forgotten the age-old system of rhythmical breathing because he doesn't understand the value of its benefits. Primitive man didn't need to learn how to breathe properly, as the physical condition of his existence made him a good breather instinctively. A child also is a good breather by instinct, but this ability is quickly lost when he becomes subjected to his modern-day environment.

To breathe through the nose is an elementary rule of correct breathing. The nose is the guardian of the inner door; its most important task is the absorption of prana from the air. You inhale through the nasal channels, which filter the air of dust particles; the air is then carried by the bronchial tubes directly to the lungs. This fresh oxygen inhaled through your nostrils is absorbed into the bloodstream and helps the blood to circulate properly. Then by exhalation through the nose again, the carbon dioxide is eliminated.

With deep breathing the diaphragm becomes strengthened and assumes proper functioning, and there is mild pressure upon the liver, stomach, and digestive tract that aids in the proper relation of the pressure in the organs in the abdomen. Our inner organs need to be exercised as well as the surface muscles.

Sports such as swimming, basketball, baseball, and tennis promote functioning of the lungs, but breathing during these activities is usually jerky and unsystematic. Thus, most of the oxygen obtained by the lungs is dissipated immediately, and one experiences a loss of energy. On the contrary, it is considered that the Yoga way of breathing refreshes you, as it has a revitalizing effect on your glands and vital organs and a calming effect on your nervous system and brain. This explains why, after practicing yoga exercises with deep breathing, you will feel rested and relaxed.

The yogis believe that the quality of the blood depends to a great extent on the quantity of oxygen absorbed by the lungs. Faulty breathing, therefore, has a direct influence on the quality of the blood, which, in turn, affects all the organs of the body.

Through deep rhythmic breathing, the intake of oxygen is greatly increased.

What "rhythmic" means:

1. Rhythm is determined by your own pulse beats. To establish your rhythm, take count of your pulse, first aloud, "One — two — three — four," repeating it a few times. Then begin to count mentally until you are absolutely sure that you have caught the rhythm of your pulse. When you begin the actual exercises, count mentally, but don't keep your attention to

it – it should become an unconscious habit.

2. Breathe through your nose by slightly contracting your throat (this will partially close the epiglottis), and keep your mouth closed. There should be a slight hissing sound coming from the back of the throat. Never raise your chest while inhaling. Your rib cage should expand on both sides. Now slowly exhale with the same hissing sound while contracting your rib cage and slightly pulling in your stomach.

3. Begin to count mentally four pulse beats while inhaling and four pulse beats while exhaling. Your breath should flow smoothly and rhythmically. "Four-in-four-out" is one exercise. Repeat five times.

After the first month increase the count to "six-in-six-out", which still counts as one exercise, and gradually add to this as you get used to additional oxygen in your system. Increase the number of exercises gradually until you reach 60 a day. Don't do them all at one time. Divide them into two or three sessions.

The Complete Yoga Breathing

Inhale, activating the diaphragm, pushing the abdomen outward. The pushing-out movement will fill the lower part of your lungs with air. This will expand the lower ribs and the middle of the thorax, gradually taking over the air from the lower part of your lungs.

Begin the exhalation, drawing the abdomen in. This lifts the diaphragm, the rib cage returns to normal position, and the air is expelled from the lungs, carrying with it the carbon dioxide from your body.

Breathe in and out smoothly, not with a jerky movement. The exhalation is also done through the nose (mouth closed). Every part of the lungs is filled with air, increasing the intake of oxygen.

CHAPTER 7: YOGA FOR WEIGHT LOSS

When you think of yoga, you might not think of it as something that is an aerobic exercise. However, yoga is a great way to lose weight and help you tone your body. By focusing on your body and the way that your muscles are moving, you are burning calories. Even though it's not an aerobic workout, it can be used to lose weight in different ways. In this chapter, I'm going to talk about how yoga can be used for weight loss and give you some recommended poses that will help with your weight loss.

Yoga is good to be used as a weight loss tool because of the psychological effects that affect the processes of the body. When you perform yoga, you are lowering your stress levels, which helps increase your insulin sensitivity, allowing your body to process fat as an energy source. So, your lower stress level will allow your body to lose weight! There is also a form of yoga that is called power yoga that is meant to be used to lose weight and gain body tone. Power yoga combines the poses of traditional yoga and makes it more of an aerobic exercise.

Since there are many yoga poses, I'm going to highlight some that are recommended for weight loss. While you might find others beneficial as well, these are the ones that are proven to help aid in burning fat. Try different poses and ways of doing yoga until you find one that works for you. Your body and mind operate differently than everyone else's so knowing what works for you is essential in finding the right routine to enhance your weight loss.

The Crescent Pose

When performing the crescent pose, you are helping to shape your abs, hips and thighs. This move has you stand with your feet together, taking a deep breath while extending your arms above your head. As you let your breath out, lower your hands to the ground. Taking another deep breath, step back with your right leg so that you're performing a lunge. Your left leg should be bent at the knee. Taking another breath, put your hands back up into the air and hold that position. Return to your original position.

Concentrating on your breathing while performing this and other yoga moves is essential to making sure that you're working your body and mind correctly.

The Willow Pose

The willow pose helps to firm the sides of your abs. In this pose, you want to raise your left leg and place it on your inner right thigh while taking a breath. When releasing your breath, extend your hands towards the sky. Lean left while taking another breath. Switch legs and repeat on the other side.

The Rocking Boat Pose

In this pose, you start seated with your feet in front of you on the ground. Lift your legs at a forty-five degree angle in front of you while taking a breath. Lean back so that you're in a v-shaped position. While breathing in and out, lessen and widen the v-shape of your body. This pose helps to tone your abs and back.

The Chair Pose

The chair pose helps tone your buttocks and thighs. In this position, you want to start with your feet shoulder width apart. Inhale while lifting your arms in front of you. While you exhale, lower yourself like you're sitting in a chair. Hold this pose for a few seconds and then return to standing position.

While these are just a few of the positions that can aid in your weight loss, try finding other ones that will benefit areas of your body that you feel need to be focused on. There are many poses out there, so find the ones that will work for you. Remember, the stress relieving effects of yoga will ultimately help you to lose weight without aerobic activity.

CHAPTER 8: PHILOSOPHY OF YOGA

Yoga is one of the six ancient schools of Hinduism, although in modern times it has often been adopted and interpreted as a secular practice. Yoga was designed and intended to be a method to logically and systematically improve yourself in all areas of body and mind. The ultimate goal of yoga is to achieve **Moksha** or release from suffering, entering a state of ultimate bliss and peace.

Yoga itself is split into numerous different schools for the purpose of achieving **Moksha,** of which four are the most prominent. These include Bhakti yoga (path of devotion), Jnana yoga (path of wisdom), Karma yoga (path of selflessness) and Raja yoga (path of mind control).

All of these different branches of yoga, can be simply called **yoga** and they all share the same aim. Nonetheless, their practices and techniques vary dramatically. Raja yoga is also known as **Ashtanga Yoga,** or eight-limbed yoga, as it involves eight steps. Occasionally, you may also hear the term 'Patanjali' yoga, which refers to the ancient Indian scholar Patanjali, who is accredited with its creation.

The eight limbs of Raja yoga are intended to be sequential and aimed to be completed one 'limb' at a time until Mohska is attained. What the West typically refers to as yoga is in fact the third limb of the eight, which is **Asanas** or postures, which often grouped under the phrase **Hatha** yoga.

The eight limbs of Raja yoga are as follows;

1) <u>Yama</u>

Yama are ethical standards for living with others, which are to be obeyed at all times. There are five yamas;

Ahisma (nonviolence)

Satya (truthfulness)

Asteya (nonstealing)

Brahmachayra (continence)

Aparigraha (concovetousness)

2) Niyama

Niyama is self-discipline and methods for spiritual living. There are five guiding principles for Niyama:

Saucha (cleanliness)

Samtosa (contentment)

Tapas (spiritual austerity)

Svadhaya (study of spirituality)

Iscara pranidhana (devotion to god)

3) Asanas

Asanas are postures, which improve strength, balance and flexibility. In yoga, the mind and the body are believed to be one. The body is a temple that must be preserved and maintained for the mind to thrive and flourish. Therefore if we fail to condition the body, all spiritual practice will be inhibited. Even if you don't belief or endorse other yoga beliefs, asanas are still useful to practice as their benefits to strength, flexibility and balance are well-documented.

4) Pranayama

Pranayama is control of the breathing. In the philosophy of yoga, the breath is associated with our energy and mood. By mastering the breathing, you are thought to be able to change your personality and invigorate your life force. Pranayama is often practiced before or after Hatha yoga and is useful to combat stress, anxiety and even depression.

5) Pratyahara

Pratyahara means withdrawal of the senses. In the yoga philosophy, transcending the senses is vital for achieving **moksha**. If we are constantly bound by the sensations around us we lack the ability to direct our attention towards ourselves, and ultimately achieve **moksha**.

6) Dharana

Dharana means concentration. Dharana is a more refined, advanced stage of awareness than our usual understanding of concentration. As the sixth limb of yoga, we have now managed to live life ethically and morally, both in our own standards and relationships with others. Our body has been strengthened, our breath is calm and steady and we have turned away from external distractions. With concentration, you start to focus upon your own mind and overcome internal distractions and thoughts.

7) Dhayana

Dhyana means meditation. With our newly found concentration, we direct our focus towards ourselves without any interruption. The difference between dhyana and dharana is effort; dhayana is involves such awareness, that you are able to monitor all sensations without needing to focus. This requires a still mind initially, but calms and stills the mind even further.

8) Samadhi

Samadhi is a state of bliss and ecstasy. When you reach samadhi, you start to transcend yourself and become connected to the divine and all other things. Samadhi is a state of great peace and joy.

This guide will focus heavily upon the **asanas** and **pranayama** in order to help you improve both body and mind. Nonetheless, it is still important to be aware of the rich context and tapestry to which both the **asanas** and **pranayama** belong. A basic understanding of the aims and structure of **Raja** yoga should help you appreciate why other people regard yoga so highly, as well as understand why specific values, such as mindfulness are regarded so highly.

CHAPTER 9: HEALTH BENEFITS OF YOGA

Yoga is a proven science that traces its origin back thousands of years and is comprised of theories and observations, which have been proven by modern science. The health benefits of yoga include control of diabetes, control of hypertension, a stronger heart, reduced back pain, relief from osteoarthritis, improvement in gastric conditions, control of asthma and bronchitis, and weight loss in a healthy way. Here are some health benefits of yoga

Daily yoga practice can bring in a number of benefits to practitioners. Yoga not only helps control diseases but also plays an important role in achieving relaxation and physical fitness.

Depression and Stress

BKS Iyengar's yoga has yogic postures for eliminating stress from the body and mind. Yogic postures such as corpse posture, child's posture, forward-bending posture, legs up the wall, cat's posture, back-bending, and headstand are considered good for eliminating depression and stress. Tests have shown positive feedback for yoga's impact on depression and stress, because participants reported a marked decrease in depression levels.

Controls Hypertension

Yoga practice and the relaxation techniques in yoga have a positive effect on blood pressure. The regular practice of postures such as shavasana, padmasana and baddha padmasana, along with pranayama techniques such as chandravedi and sheetali, help in reducing blood pressure. These postures keep the body and mind in a relaxed state. A study on yoga's role in controlling blood pressure showed more positive results compared to the placebo treatments.

Yoga for a Healthy Heart

Yoga and a change in lifestyle can help in keeping a healthy heart and body. Ujjayi pranayama and bhramari pranayama are beneficial for the heart. Other postures such as vajrasana, janushirasana, padahastasana and baddha padmasana, along with pranayama techniques like sarala pranayama and Chandra bhedi pranayama can be practiced for a healthier body. A study on people with coronary artery diseases showed that by including yoga in their normal routine, as well as a lifestyle change and a healthy diet, the incidence of coronary artery disease was reduced drastically.

Diabetes Control

Regular yoga practice can also help in controlling diabetes. Some of the postures that can aid in controlling diabetes include pavanamuktasana, ardhamatsyendrasana, gomukhasana, koormasana, bhujangasana, dhanurasana, and mayurasana. Apart from these postures, pranayama exercises such as suryabhedi, ujjayi and bhastrika have also been prescribed for diabetes. Controlled tests on diabetic patients resulted in improved diabetic conditions for the majority of people who had undergone some sort of yoga training.

Back Pain Relief

Yoga may benefit individual's with lower back pain as well. Some yoga poses or postures, such as mountain pose, pigeon pose, wall plank pose, back traction, and child's posture, can provide relief from lower back pain.

Stomach Disorders

Gastric troubles can be relieved by practicing yoga. Certain asanas, or postures such as pavanamuktasana, padahastasana, and padangusthasana help in controlling gastric troubles, tone up abdominal muscles, increase gastric juices, and improve digestion. These postures are simple forward-bending postures where one has to touch one's feet without bending the knees and take it forward to an extent that the palms must come under his or her feet with ease. This can help you feel relief from a wide variety of gastrointestinal issues.

Osteoarthritis Relief

Yoga works well in controlling musculo skeletal pain as well, especially osteoarthritis. The efficacy of yoga on osteoarthritis was studied on people suffering from osteoarthritis in hands. The tests showed that practicing yoga is effective in providing relief from hand osteoarthritis.

Asthma and Bronchitis

Pranayama, or breathing exercises, in yoga are good for asthma patients. Yoga postures such as half-spinal twist, wind-relieving posture, and corpse posture, along with alternating nostril breathing technique can act as remedies for asthma and bronchitis.

Carpal Tunnel Syndrome

Carpal tunnel syndrome is a condition characterized by pressure on the nerves in the wrist. These nerves supply feeling and movement in the hand. This condition causes weakness, numbness, and tingling and may also cause muscle damage in the hand or fingers. Yoga can reduce the effects of carpal tunnel syndrome significantly.

Increases Flexibility

There are specific yoga postures that positively affect various joints and stress points of the body. Yoga enhances lubrication of these joints, ligaments, and tendons, making them flexible and functional.

Detoxification

Yoga ensures gentle stretching of muscles and joints, along with the comprehensive workout of various internal organs, which in turn improves the optimum blood supply. A healthy blood flow is essential in flushing out the toxins and providing nourishment to every cell in the body for a zestful life. Yoga can slacken the pace of aging and ensure vitality.

Chapter 10: Losing Weight Through Yoga

Regularly practicing yoga can certainly help make you feel better about your body. It increases your strength, makes you more flexible and helps tone your muscles as well. However, many people do use it as a means of safely losing weight. Not a lot of people are aware of the fact that yoga can help you shed any excess pounds you may have put on. However, does it really work?

The thing that most beginners need to know about losing weight through yoga is the fact that there are many different varieties of it. There are lighter varieties of the practice designed to calm the body and clear the mind. Whilst these can help in some way, you need to practice them in conjunction with other forms of exercise such as jogging, walking and aerobics. Of course, a healthy diet is a must as well.

You can also find vigorous forms of yoga that can provide you with a better workout if your ultimate goal is to lose weight. These are more advanced forms of the practice and before you start doing them, it is recommended that you go through the basics first. In doing so, you can help minimize the risk of injuries.

The most athletic yoga styles fall under the vinyasa or flow category. These styles start with fast-paced poses known as "sun salutation" which is then followed by a steady flow of standing poses. This style will keep you moving. As you get warmer, backbends and deeper stretches are introduced. Some of the most popular Vinyasa styles of yoga include:

☐**Ashtanga:** This particular type of yoga is very vigorous and its practitioners are often the most dedicated yogis. If you are a beginner, it is highly encouraged that you sign up for group classes as this would help motivate you to continue practicing it. The series of poses are quite easy to learn and once you are familiar with them, you can take your practice at home.

Poses:

The primary series is what is often referred to as the Yoga Chikitsa. It is intended to help in realigning the spine, build strength, detoxify the body as well as boost stamina and flexibility. This is a series comprised of about 75 poses and usually takes an hour or two to complete, depending on how familiar you are with it.

The next series is referred to as the Nadi Shodana and it helps with strengthening as well as cleansing the nervous system, along with all the other subtle energy channels in our body. The last four series, also considered as more advanced yoga varieties, are called Sthira Bhaga. This means divine stability and focuses more on difficult arm balances that require a lot of practice should beginners try and attempt to perform them.

For the most part, people do skip this particular stage in the progression but if you're keen on both improving your level as a yogi and getting the workout that you need then you can give it a try.

Is Ashtanga right for you? Whilst it is quite popular, attracting students from all levels of the practice because of its athletic and vigorous style, it certainly is not meant for everyone. Trying it should help you assess if the poses are something you can pull off. The style appeals, particularly, to those who prefer doing this independently and who appreciate a sense of order in how they work.

☐**Power Yoga:** This refers to a fitness-based approach to the traditional Vinyasa style of yoga. Often referred to as "gym yoga", the practice was actually molded after the Ashtanga method but differs in that power yoga does not follow a set series of poses. This can make every class unique and keeps things interesting for the practitioner. It places emphasis on improving strength as well as flexibility, with weight loss being a common result of regular practice as well.

The style can range from gentle stretching to more intense, flowing styles. This dynamic can really give the body quite the workout and certainly provides the more athletic people with a challenge.

Is power yoga for you? The practice can vary from one teacher to the other and more often than not, it appeals to the people who are already physically fit. However, if you are keen on challenging yourself whilst losing weight, this might be the right fit. There are minimal amounts of meditation and chanting when it comes to power yoga so if you are only looking for action then this is the practice for you.

☐**Hot Yoga:** This particular type of yoga refers to classes done in a heated room. The temperature is often maintained at around 95 to 100 degrees, providing practitioners with a continuous and even warmth throughout the entire session. Typically, hot yoga follows a vinyasa style of movement wherein the instructor provides students with a series of linked poses to follow. The added element of heat actually makes this one of the more vigorous yoga sessions and certainly helps when it comes to weight loss.

Is hot yoga right for you? Many people tend to ask this question, considering the fact that this particular style of yoga is quite vigorous compared to other forms. The answer depends on your preferences and abilities. Given the additional element of heat, you may want to start slow and leave hot yoga for later. This should allow you to gradually move up and prepare yourself as the poses get more advanced.

Alright, so now that we've covered the basics of the three best yoga varieties for weight loss, let's take a closer look at each and go through some of the fundamental poses to help you get started!

CHAPTER 11: GET FLEXIBLE

Before starting many of the yoga exercises, like downward dog, you will want to get flexible. Yoga will require the use of various muscles that you may not have used recently. It will depend greatly on the type of exercising you have been doing in recent months. The information in this section will assume you have not been getting enough exercise and will need to build your strength and flexibility for more challenging yoga moves.

You should understand swimming, running and walking can be an enjoyable exercise for cardio, but yoga is not cardio related. It is about flexibility and relaxation, with many of the positions based on strengthening muscles. If you are not prone to stretching your muscles, keeping them active, and remaining flexible, you want to start with the information in this section.

Even if you do strength training, there are still several poses that will test your muscles in different ways to help you gain all-around strength versus increasing the strength of only certain muscles.

If you have not tried to touch your toes, stretch your arms behind your back, or over your chest, then you will want to go slowly. Yoga is about repetition, but two or three reps, once per week for a few weeks and then increasing to two to four times per week, will help you regain the flexibility you had as a child. You can even become more flexible than you were at a younger age. It is all dependent on the dedication you put into training your body.

Step 1: Gentle Yoga Stretches for Flexibility

You will need to start with the exercise in chapter one, to get your mind and body relaxed; therefore, open to the yoga positions you need to be in.

Once you feel your mind is open and your body relaxed, move your right leg into a bent position.

Lift your arms, to wrap your hands around your knee.

Pull gently towards you, while leaving your left leg stretched on the floor, with your toes pointing at the ceiling.

Only move your right leg as far as it is comfortable. You want to feel the muscles pull in your left leg, but you do not want to feel pain. Hold the position for the count of 8.

Switch the positions of your left and right leg. Repeat the process with the left leg.

You will switch from right to left, three times.

Step 2: Adding your Abdomen Muscles

After you have stretched your legs three times, it will be time to add an abdominal muscle stretch. With this exercise, you will again bring your right knee up as far as you can, without straining your muscles.

The additional move to this yoga position is to lift from the abdomen, moving your head and chest closer to your knee. Hold it for eight counts. Let your back fall gently back to the floor, extend your head and neck, then let your right leg extend back to the resting position.

Repeat this move with your left leg.

Switch legs three times each, while extending your head and chest towards your knee, and then along the floor.

For breathing, you always want to exhale as you move your knee to your chest and when you lift your upper body using your abdominal muscles. Breathe in and out naturally as you hold the position, then exhale as you let go.

Both stretches are working on your leg muscles. You may feel they are tight at first, with a partial split of your legs. The extended leg will often feel tight on the inside of the thigh, while your muscles running through the knee from your buttocks will feel tight as you pull your leg closer to your abdomen.

When you add the back lift from the abdominal muscles, you will feel the muscles in your back, shoulders and neck tighten. You should always stop if you feel pain and try extending less when pain results.

Move slowly through the repetitions to avoid hurting your muscles; particularly, if you have not stretched in several months.

Step 3: Gaining Flexibility in your Upper Body

Flexibility is just as important for your upper body as it is for your lower body. To gain more flexibility you need all of your muscles to stretch without causing you pain. If you have pain anywhere in your muscles, it is linked to improper stretching or not stretching at all. When you start exercising after an extended period, you may not have the flexibility you once did. There is the possibility of harming your muscles, such as tearing a ligament.

There are exercises you learned in school, such as touching your toes to stretch out your back and leg muscles. In yoga, you can do these same stretches to help with your back. You can also roll your neck to loosen it up but, ultimately, what provides the best medicine for your body will be the relaxation, breathing and use of simple poses that help you maintain the flexibility you are building in this section.

For your upper body, begin with mountain pose. It may seem like a mundane, unhelpful pose but, in reality, it is the start to many poses that will help you gain balance, peace of mind and flexibility.

Mountain pose requires you to stand with your feet together on a yoga mat. Make sure your entire foot is on the floor, with your hands at your sides. You will want to center your head and upper body over your hips. Maintain this position for one count before lifting up, without moving your feet. You are raising from your flat feet, through your muscles, up your spine, and through your head to be in a centered position. You want to elongate your spine, so you are standing up completely straight without slouching. Your arms are extended, fully, to the fingertips. During Mountain pose, breathe easily, in and out. Repeat three times to start off with. Then, as you use these exercises to warm up for other yoga poses, add five more repetitions.

Step 4: Chair

Beginning with Mountain pose, raise your arms over your head, reaching through your fingertips. Sit back and down as if there is a chair behind you. This will change the weight to your heels while extending your abdomen. Chair pose helps strengthen your legs, upper back and shoulders. It also helps with flexibility because you are using different muscles to those you used while on the floor. Your arms are meant to assist you in balance.

Start with a three times repetition before increasing to eight reps per session. It is a warm-up move that will help you as you complete it eight times. You can even build on the eight repetitions by creating three sets of eight movements.

Step 5: Modified Downward Facing Dog

Before you move into one of the best yoga poses, the Downward Facing Dog, you will need the flexibility, strength and balance to master it. A modified Downward Facing Dog will use a chair. The chair back should be waist height. You will place your hands on the back of the chair. Your palms need to face down, with your fingertips outstretched, and your arms need to be shoulder width apart. Step your feet back until they are perfectly aligned with your hips. Your body will look like a right angle with the chair. Your spine needs to be parallel to the floor, while your feet are flat and your legs are straight. You should feel a burn through your legs, specifically in the hamstrings. Your head should be parallel to your spine. The shoulders and upper arms will be open, helping to stretch the spine, without placing weight on your upper body.

Step 6: Bound Angle

For this pose, you are going to sit on the ground. It is one of flexibility and can be done in a few different ways. First, make certain your hips are straight with your spine. Keep your shoulders open. You can begin by keeping your legs straight in front of you. You do not want them in a Buddha pose or cross-legged pose. Bring your legs up to the knees, bending with your feet flat on the ground. Once your legs are bent, open at the hips by turning out your legs into a butterfly position, with the soles of your feet together. For balance, place your arms, with your hands flat on the yoga mat, behind you. Your hands should have the fingertips facing behind you with your inner arms turned forward. Your neck and spine should remain in alignment. Hold this pose for thirty seconds each time. You will feel a burn in your groin area and inner thighs until you gain more flexibility.

Yoga is about strengthening your muscles, as well as achieving better balance and flexibility. As you move through more challenging poses, you will see more flexibility occurring in your body. There are certain poses that you will want to modify if you have yet to regain flexibility. This is possible, often, by bending your knees slightly to lessen the strain on your leg muscles.

Step 7: Downward Facing Dog

You have already used a modified pose for Downward Facing Dog. The hope is that you will not move on to this strengthening exercise until you are more flexible. However, if necessary bend at the knee slightly to take some of the weight off the leg muscles. Start by putting your feet shoulder width apart.

Bend at the waist and touch the floor. From this position walk your hands out in front of you, until your feet feel as if they will lift from the ground. You want to keep your feet flat on the mat. Your arms need to be straight, with your head and spine aligned. You are going to create a triangle with your body. Two sides are your body, and the third is the floor. Your weight should be evenly distributed. One thing that many new yoga practitioners do is put all their weight on their hands. You should not do this. You are not bending your wrists at a ninety-degree angle. Rather, your wrists should only bend slightly to keep your palms on the floor. Your weight should be evenly distributed between your feet and arms. This pose helps increase strength in your arms and leg muscles since they are supporting you.

Step 8: Bridge

The bridge is a simple abdominal strengthening exercise. It requires you to lie on the ground. Lie flat on your yoga mat, with your hands by your sides, palms facing up. Make sure your spine is aligned, and your neck is stretched. Bring your feet up together, bending at the knees. Lift your mid-body from the knees and shoulders. Your shoulders and feet should remain on the ground while you create a bridge with your body. You are going to stretch your spine and neck, but also increase your abdominal muscles with the move because you are relying on your stomach muscles to help you keep the position in line.

Step 9: Plank

The plank is one of the most challenging poses for someone who has weak wrists or uses their hands a lot. This pose is not recommended if you have carpal tunnel syndrome or arthritis. It places a lot of weight on your hands and wrists. You will begin in Downward Facing Dog, walking your legs backward to move your heels off the mat. In plank, your entire spine is straight, with your head and neck aligned. You are going to bend at the wrists at a 90-degree angle, keeping your arms straight. Your toes will support your legs. This position is ideal for abdominal strength because you need to keep your body in a perfectly straight position while bending at the toes and wrists. It is a great pose for core strength and balance.

Step 10: Chaturanga Dandasana

This is a modified plank pose, with more difficulty. Again, if you have trouble in your hands and wrists, this pose is not recommended. The difference with Chaturanga Dandasana is the bent elbows. Your upper arms will be in perfect parallel alignment with your spine, while your hands are flat on the ground, and your wrists are bent at 90-degrees, for your lower arms to support you. Your toes are also going to keep your legs off the ground. Your body will be parallel to the floor, with no knees bent. You will hold this pose for at least eight seconds. It is all about core stability and strengthening of your triceps and abdominal muscles; however, it also puts much of your weight on your hands and toes.

Step 11: Upward Facing Dog

In this pose, you move from Chaturanga Dandasana to Upward Facing Dog. Your toes will no longer be bent, but straight on the floor, with the tops of your feet touching the mat. You are going to push up with your arms, straightening the bent elbows, while bending at the waist, backward to look up at the ceiling. You are bending backward instead of forwards in this pose. It helps to open your chest and shoulders, while also stretching the abdomen in a back position.

CHAPTER 13: TYPES OF YOGA

There are several different types of yoga. Most people just think of yoga as being one standard set of poses, but it's not quite that simple.Western yoga is generally just defined as "yoga". There aren't usually any types mentioned. Western yoga often uses a mixture of different yoga types, and different instructors may even come up with their own poses or mix their own unique blends.There are in fact six types of yoga traditionally practiced, plus a new type, bikram yoga, that has been rapidly gaining in popularity recently.

The six traditional types of yoga are:

Hatha

Raja

Karma

Bhakti

Jnana

Tantra

Now we're going to take a closer look at each individual types of yoga and their differences.Hatha Yoga. The teachings of hatha yoga are the type most commonly practiced in the Western hemisphere. The word hatha comes from the Sanskrit term ha (meaning sun).There are two important principles that hatha yoga is based on:

Meditation – You will find at least one posture that is especially comfortable to you and that you can sustain for long period of time while you meditate. As you advance, you'll ideally learn several postures that you are comfortable with. Many people find the lotus position especially helpful for meditation.

Improving Energy Within The Body – This is all about improving the flow of energy throughout your body so improve your overall health.

Raja Yoga

Raja yoga is very similar to hatha yoga. Raja is considered a bit more difficult than other forms of yoga, because it requires more discipline and control than other forms.

Raja yoga focuses on concentration, meditation, and discipline of the mind and body. There are eight limbs of raja yoga:

Moral discipline

Self restraint

Concentration

Meditation

Breath control

Posture

Sensory inhibition

Ecstasy (not the drug!)

Karma Yoga

The word karma means "action". Karma is generally thought of as the unseen force in the world that causes good things to happen to good people and bad things to pay back those who have done wrong. Karma yoga means selfless action. To perform karma yoga, you are supposed to surrender yourself completely to serve the greater good - the good of man and humanity.The founder of karma yoga is Bhagavad Vita. This version is heavily rooted in Hinduism. Although you don't have to practice Hinduism to practice karma yoga, you should potentially familiarize yourself with the teachings of Hinduism in order to fully understand and appreciate karma yoga.

Bhakti Yoga

Bhatki yoga is a sensual, erotic form of yoga. It's all about love, divine love, specifically.Love operates on three levels according the principles of bhatki yoga:

Material love

Human love

Spiritual love

Jnana Yoga

Jnana yoga is all about wisdom and enlightenment. It's about clearing the mind and the soul and releasing negativity. It's about transformation and taking the path to true enlightenment.

Tantra Yoga

Tantra yoga is perhaps the type of yoga people are most curious about. It's not about sex exclusively, but that is a part of it. It is about reaching enlightenment and transcending the self through several rituals. Sex is indeed one of those rituals, but it is not the only one by any means. Some tantric practitioners even recommend a life of celibacy. Tantra means "expansion". The aim of tantra yoga is to expand your mind so that you can reach all levels of consciousness. It uses rituals to bring out the male and female aspects within an individual in order to awake the true spirit within.

Bikram Yoga

Bikram yoga is a relatively new form of yoga. It is not included in the six traditional forms of yoga, but it is becoming so popular it deserves a very special mention. Bikram yoga was developed by Bikram Choudhury. It takes place in a room that is at 105°F with a humidity of about 40%. There are 26 postures and two types of breathing exercises.Bikram yoga is more about detoxifying the body rather than reaching some sort of spiritual enlightenment. By forcing the body to sweat profusely, toxins are eliminated through the skin. Additionally, the extra warmth makes the body more flexible, which helps prevent injury, relieves stress, and helps aid in deeper stretching. Some people oppose Bikram yoga because it defeats the very principles of yoga. It has been heavily commercialized, and its creators protect it by copyright.

CHAPTER 14: UNDERSTANDING YOGA- YOGA FOR THE ULTIMATE BEGINNER

While you may already know the meaning of yoga, I find that it helps to start with the meaning first so that we can be on the same page, especially because the understanding of Yoga is often times marred by many misunderstandings.

Yoga is a Sanskrit word that means Listen. Yoga is a terminology and a blanket for the whole practice of Yoga that includes philosophy, religion, and practice. In addition to the popular physical practice and disciplines of Yoga (referred to as Hatha Yoga), there is more to Yoga than meets the eyes. Let us get an understanding of the practice before embarking on our journey.

As a practice, Yoga is mental, spiritual, and physical discipline. A person who practices yoga is referred to as a Yogi, and as most yogis will tell you, the main aim of yoga is to transform the mind and body. Yoga as a term signifies a number of practices, schools, and goals. For instance, in Buddhism, Jainism, and Hinduism, the most popular form of Yoga is the Raja yoga and the Hatha yoga that we shall look at later.

It may also interest you to learn that yoga literally means yoking together, which is a span of oxen or horses. The term was later applied to mean the 'yoking' together of the mind and body. Some people (actually, most people) may also be wondering about the origins of yoga as a practice. There is speculation that the practice of yoga dates back to pre-Vedic Indian tradition. However, the general understanding is that the practice developed around the 5th and 6th centuries BCE. If we were to go into the specifics, the earliest accounts of the practice are in the Buddhist Nikayas, with parallel development recorded in the Yoga Sutras of Patanjali around 400 CE. As far as speculation goes, the popular Hatha yoga did not come into being until the turn of the first millennium. There is also an understanding amongst yogis that Hatha yogi developed from tantra.

Today's practice of yoga in most western countries including the U.S and the UK dates back to the late 19th and 20th century where yoga gurus from India introduced it after the success of Swami Vivekananda (An Indian Hindu monk). Prior to the 1980's, Yoga was not very popular as a physical exercise across the world or the western world except in India. This form of physical yoga exercise is what is often times known as Hatha yoga that gained popularity after the 80's.

The philosophies of yoga dictate that humans consist of three bodies, the physical, the subtle, and the casual. It goes further to state that the body also consists of five sheets namely the food sheet, the prana-breath, intellect, the bliss, and the mind sheet. All the above cover the atman (self or human body), the energy, and their channels that are all concentrated on chakras (energy centers in the body). While this may all be very fascinating, it does not really explain why you should practice yoga. Recent studies have proven that yoga is very useful as a contemporary intervention for ailments such as schizophrenia, heart disease, asthma, and cancer. Nevertheless, this is not all; here are a few more reasons why you should practice yoga.

Why you should practice yoga?

Most of us have very different reasons why we practice this beautiful art known as yoga. Contrary to popular belief and despite the fact that toning the body is a central part of yoga, there is more to it than that. For one, yoga goes beyond the physical and into the mental and spiritual. Here is another surprising fact for you; yoga also helps detoxify your body. Your reasons for practicing yoga may vary from mine, but here are some fundamental reasons why yoga is an ideal form of exercise not only for your body, but also for your spirituality and mental wellness.

P.s. Despite the fact that 80% of all yogis are women, yoga is ideal for any human, male or female. (We shall only cover five important reasons because you are most probably aware of the benefits of yoga).

Pack the stress in shipping boxes

When most people hear this about yoga, they think that it is simply media hype; they could not be more wrong. Yoga is the ultimate stress reliever. We all have different ways of managing stress; some of us would rather go to the gym and punch out our stress and furry at the punching bag (which ends up increasing your aggressiveness and tiredness), while some of us prefer to binge eat. While all these methods may seem to work, they are not long-term solutions because they have negative effects. Enter yoga; yoga is neither aggressive nor passive. It combines relaxation techniques that if practiced regularly, have a very calming effect. How so? Because, on top of training your body i.e. body muscles, yoga also has a mental and spiritual component to it that helps the mind to see the bigger picture and thus act intuitively rather than acting out (freaking out). In addition, the time you allocate to yoga i.e. unplug from the frantic world of calls, IM, texts, and emails, you get some time to yourself and thus reflect on your future and your overall wellbeing.

Improves flexibility

Do you remember those praying mantis poses we talked about at the beginning of this book? They are part of the beauty of yoga. Sure, they do not come easy, but once you get started, you will never want to look back. Most physical postures of yoga are inclusive of at least one spinal twist; this is to loosen the many joints that make up the spine. Stretching the spine is the ultimate strength and energy boost any athlete or non-athlete needs. It can greatly improve our back swing or tennis game as well as improve other parts of your life including the bedroom. Flexibility from the practice of yoga can also greatly improve the body's ability to digest food and detoxification, which improve the body's health and immune system.

Have Chiseled muscles (the crux of the practice)

Are you wondering how "praying mantis" stretches and poses make your muscles stronger? Here is how; by using your body weight. This sounds very ambiguous, but there is a lot of truth to it. Let me ask you a question; how many free weights does it take you to bench press your body? Well, yoga allows you the same without the weights by combining a series of pushups, leg lifts and squats to chisel out your body muscles. The results are biceps and triceps worth the name 'guns' and muscles that are the envy of any muscle or toned body enthusiast.

Injury free exercise

Anyone who has worked out in the gym will tell you that the fingers of one hand are not enough to count the number of injuries they have sustained in the gym.

Yoga classes on the other hand commence with the lesson that your first goal is to honor your body needs on any particular day. While this may not be the ultimate exercise injury remedy, it helps you realize your daily limitations, as well as equipping you with the skills to assess your body. This helps reduce the risk of injury. Additionally, the yoga stretches and poses you perform help you reduce the risk of injury as you undertake other forms of exercise such as running because the joints in use are already flexible from the practice.

Better sex

If you look at the pages of the Kama sutra, you will quickly notice that some of the poses in the book are near impossible for the average Mary and Joe. You can translate all those "praying mantis yoga poses" directly into the bedroom. Additionally, the breathing and relaxation techniques in yoga are transferable into the bedroom for longer and better sex. Because of your strengthened concentration, energy and core muscles, you can better focus your sexual energy. This can prove very helpful especially for men who are prone to premature ejaculation and for women because the core strength exercises can also help them stretch their vagina muscles for explosive orgasms.

Yoga is also the ultimate glowing skin remedy. How so? Do you remember all that detoxification that yoga can help your body perform? It translates directly into a radiant skin tone! In addition, all the amazing sex you will have as your expertise in yoga increases will have an effect on your body including, the skin.

The Different Types of Yoga Explained

Now that we have seen the wonderful effects yoga can have on your body and life, it is only right that we go a little deeper by looking at the types of yoga there are. Remember that the most commonly practiced type of yoga is the Hatha. This does not mean that its practice is the epitome of a true yogi; there is much more to yoga than any novice or expert can fathom. Let us look at the types of yoga to gain a better understanding of the practice.

Types of yoga

1-Anusara

An American yogi who goes by the name John Friend developed Anusara yoga in 1997. This makes Anusara a relative newcomer in the realms of yoga practice. The practice of Anusara relies heavily on the doctrine that we (all humans) are full of intrinsic goodness. The practice therefore aims to use the physical part of yoga to help the practitioner open up their heart and be open to the experience of grace and thus let their goodness shine through each and every part of their life. The classes, all based on the principle of alignment are involved and rigorous and thus must be under the guidance of a teacher especially in the initial stages of practice but the benefits to the body and mind are unfathomable.

2-Ashtanga

If you are looking for a yoga technique with traditional yoga techniques as its bedrock, then Ashtanga is your best shot. Although it is based on traditional teachings, its introduction into the west was by Pattabhi Jois, which is pronounced as "Pah-tah-bee Joyce" in the 70's. Similar to the Anusara, the Ashtanga is rigorous and follows specific sequenced postures that are similar to the Vinyasa yoga. Each style and pose in this type of yoga links to each breath with the main difference in the Ashtanga being that you have to perform the exact poses in the exact order always. This type of yoga is very demanding (mentally and physically), which makes it the ideal choice for anyone looking to develop their core muscles and body strength.

3-Bikram

Bikram Choudhury is the "father" of this type of yoga, with the initial introduction being approximately 30 years ago. Classes for this type of yoga happen in heated rooms. If you are looking to let out some sweat in your yoga sessions, there is not better choice than this type of yoga. The classes consist of 26 poses that always follow the same sequence (much like the Ashtanga, albeit being different). While the practice of yoga is not often times controversial, Bikram is because of the trademark filled by Choudhury that has led him to sue studios that teach Bikram contrary to the sequence and poses exactly as he says they should. Despite this, Bikram is very popular perhaps because he describes the poses and sequence very well and thus they are easier to perform compared to other types of Yoga.

4-Hatha

Hatha yoga is a term that describes, or refers to any type of yoga that teaches any physical yoga pose. This makes it the most

102

popular type of yoga mainly because almost every type of yoga practiced in most western countries falls here. By labelling a yoga class as a hatha class, it means that the first few classes will consist mainly of an introduction to basic yoga poses. Hatha yoga is not your typical "sweat kiln" yoga and you should not expect to work up a sweat while practicing it. However, you gain a lot of from its practice and I can guarantee that you will leave your yoga class feeling relaxed and looser than you have ever felt.

5-Hot Yoga

Hot yoga is profoundly similar to Bikram albeit a little different. The main difference between the two is that the poses in hot yoga vary from those in Bikram. Hot yoga is ideal for those of us who want to work up a sweat as we maneuver our way through intricate poses and the breathing techniques. The yoga studio in hot yoga will be hot just like in Bikram.

6-Iyengar

The correct pronunciation for this is "eye-yen-gar." B.K.S Iyengar developed and popularized it. If you want to be meticulous in your yoga pose and practice, Iyengar is the way to go. The style pays very close attention to finding the correct pose and alignment. A typical Iyengar studio will stock different yoga props such as blankets, bolsters, chairs, rope wall, blocks etc., all with one agenda; to help you find the proper alignment. An Iyengar class is also not your typical "sweat kiln" because there is very little jumping around. However, the classes are immensely challenging, mentally and physically. An Iyengar teacher undergoes thorough and comprehensive training before certification. This type of yoga is ideal if you suffer from a chronic condition or have an injury and is most likely the best form of yoga due to the stringency of its training and certification that ensures you have a qualified teacher.

7-Restorative

When you want to relax, restorative yoga is your best choice. Classes in this type of yoga use blankets, bolsters, blocks etc. to help the practitioner (you) into passive poses. This forces the body into a relaxed pose without necessarily putting in the effort. In fact, most practitioners of this type of yoga claim that a restorative yoga class is more relaxing and rejuvenating than a power nap. In most western countries, the classes mostly occur on Friday evenings and nights when most people need the rest after a long week.

8-Vinyasa

The correct pronunciation for this is "Vin-yah-Sah." In Sanskrit, it means flow. This means that most of their classes are fluid in their nature with practices that are very movement intense. A typical Vinyasa class will have a teacher who choreographs his moves and poses to transition from pose to pose with some soft music playing in the background to keep the rhythm going. Vinyasa is very intensive and similar to Ashtanga; however, the classes in Vinyasa do not follow a specific pattern, and thus each class is different. This type of yoga is ideal for those of us who hate routine and love to test our limit, physical and mental.

9-Kundalini yoga

The main reasoning behind the development of kundalini yoga is to awaken energies in the spine. A typical kundalini class will involve some yoga, breathing techniques and mediation, as well as some chanting, and something called the alternate nostril breathing.

10- Yin Yoga

This type of yoga is passive in nature. It comes from a Taoist tradition and uses seated postures to target tissues in the lower spine, pelvis, and hips. This type of yoga advocates for poses that are held from anywhere between a minute to ten minutes once the practitioner gets into the pose. The poses all have one main goal; to encourage "letting go" and increase flexibility. For the complete yoga beginner, this is the absolute first step because it teaches basic meditation techniques that help you still the mind. It is also the ideal go to technique for athletes looking for tension release in joint and for those of us looking for an ideal way to relax.

It is also important to note that despite covering all major types of yoga in this chapter, I have left out many more. It is also important to note that all we have learnt in this chapter may be different when you visit a yoga studio. How so? Because of the similarity between the poses in most of the types of yoga, most yogis (teachers) will use the different types of yoga poses and types together to strike a good balance in all the parts of the body. This means that while you may want to learn a specific type of yoga, learning that type may also mean gaining experience in all the other types because most of the poses in all of them are very similar except in some types of yoga that are more demanding than others are.

We have covered just about everything there is to learn before getting into the practice of the art. We shall now look into some of the poses that you can practice even at home without your teacher.

CHAPTER 15: WHY BREATHING IS IMPORTANT FOR YOGA

'Ayama' growth indicates an extension. It also identifies the breath and the life force's discipline. Pranic flow is lengthened by the discipline through the body. We spread the pranic energy into ourselves affecting the brain and the blood. Our aim is thus, to control the prana entering our anatomies to control your brain. Pranayama's practice retains the body in radiant health. Concentration and focus are restored.

Pranayama must be practiced through the nose. Many don't breath correctly. The average person breathes utilizing the leading portion of the lung. They avoid using the diaphragm and breathe through the mouth. This causes reduced strength as a limited amount of vital atmosphere is taken in. Its set up in a way to get a lower resistance to infection. The lungs are not flushed properly of all stale air. When we breathe through the nose, we filter and warm the air entering our systems. The breath travels through the olfactory organs, which lie at the back of the nose. Prana is therefore, in reach of the central nervous system along with the brain.

Nasal breathing is utilized during yoga asanas.

One maintains the mouth breaths deeply, breathing prana completing the leading portion, middle and bottom part of the lung and shut. The abdomen expands around the inhalation. The diaphragm moves along, which then massages the abdominal organs.

Together with the exhalation, the diaphragm, and the belly agreements progress. The heart gets a good massage out of this movement. This can be opposite from the way many are used to breathing and does take exercise. The easiest way is to always observe ones inhaling alternately or look into a mirror when lying down or sitting up, set your hand on your stomach to feel its movement.

There are three periods with any yoga asana, as to pranayama;

Breathing or 'parka' ensures the practitioner breathes in pranic vitality to complete the lungs,

Exhalation or 'rich aka' could be the next period. You've got to exhale all of the old air to ensure that there is enough space for a great deal of excellent, energy that is vital to entering.

Preservation or 'kumbhaka' is the third level. Preservation is approximately holding the oxygen in the body before exhaling.

Remember to not stress while practicing Pranayama. Pressure causes the body to tense, which in turn causes the air to speed up, evoking the heart to beat faster. The deep breathing is then moved. Pranayama is usually to be used in a comfortable environment. You've got to be in a setting that is not too cool or too hot. The body needs to be free of stress. The mind and the body will relax. When exercising, we observe our personal rhythm. One's heart beats slower once we are comfortable. Whenever we are puzzled, stressed or anxious, one's heart beats faster and more unpredictable. The key is to be mindful and informed of the breathing.

The exercise of Pranayama is of crucial importance. The viewing of the kinds of breathing can refresh one of the much-needed energy. So do adults just like a baby requires naptime. The training of breath is that naptime. Once you're 'alert' you'll be as restored and rejuvenated like a baby, ready to target.

Easy Pranayama Exercise

This is a simple breathing exercise one could follow which doesn't involve a Yoga Guru's help.

Come to a pose. Stay put, having the spine straight.

Sit on the ground or in an upright seat. Don't choose a soft chair.

Take a few great breaths and after that come to focus.

While hearing the breath, produce the noise 'So' on breathing and then 'Pig' on exhalation internally with the mouth closed. This means 'the heart am I.' Blessings can be good when making this rule. The doctor recognizes that God's greatness is within you.

When exhaling, make the sound of the water. This provides consciousness to the air and helps constrict the flow of the breath.

Be conscious of the actual movement of your body, the surge, and drop of the belly.

Practice this Pranayama exercise for approximately 15minutes.

One prepares with correct deep pranayama for meditation. Meditation is not the lack of thought; it is somewhat the enjoying, viewing of all views that enter your brain then taking the ideas of one right into a single-focus.

Chapter 16: Why Yoga Is Best For Stress Management

Studies have shown that doing yoga leads to lower blood pressure and reduced levels of cortisol or the "stress hormone." It is also an effective form of hormone therapy as it helps regulate and stimulate the production of chemicals throughout the endocrine system.

Yoga relieves tension through moves that help increase flexibility and relax the kinks and tightness you might feel in your muscles and bones. This also leads to improved strength and balance.

It helps the body slow down and be more in tune with the universe. There is much emphasis on the connection of the body to the mind and spirit. This changes the way you view the world, where you no longer focus on the things you cannot control. Most yoga poses can only be successfully done if you learn to let go of doubts, fears and frustrations. Such is the power of yoga on managing stress and the rest of your life.

The forward bend is a simple yet effective way of exploring your body's limits. You can do a forward bend sitting ("Paschimottanasana") or standing up ("Uttanasana"). Essentially, you are folding your torso forward towards your legs and reaching your toes. If you are tense and tight, this would be more difficult to accomplish. It is not a matter of pushing yourself to fold forward, thereby stressing your muscles. You will find that when your muscles are relaxed, a forward bend is easier to do. Stay in this pose for as long as you like, simply being mindful of your breathing.

"ViparitaKarani" or the legs-up-the-wall pose is great for stress reduction and is believed to slow down ageing. The asana sends blood back to your heart, and in doing so, renews it. You can do this by lying on your mat placed beside a wall. Spread your arms out to your side. Raise your legs and prop them up on the wall. Adjust your position so your legs form a 90-degree angle with your torso. A more advanced version of this inversion is the "Sarvangasana" or a shoulder stand, where you prop your hips up with your hands. Your elbows are rooted on the ground. You will be able to raise your legs up to the sky without the support of a wall.

"UttanaShishosana" or The Puppy Pose is a heart-opening asana that counters the slouching we usually develop from hunching over a computer, sitting at a desk all day, or any type of "back-breaking" work that leads to stress. Begin kneeling on your mat, then reach your arms up and forward followed by your torso. Keep your chest lifted from the floor with your arms planted on the mat.

CHAPTER 17:20 COMMON YOGA POSES AND THEIR BENEFITS

It is important that you first take into consideration factors like your skills and limitations before you start practicing yoga. In case you have injuries in your back or poor balance, aim to start slow and then gently stretch yourself. Also, ensure that you wear loose fitting clothes and are not extremely full as this will affect your ability to do these yoga poses.

1. Mountain or Tadasana

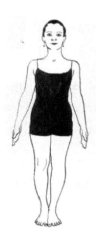

This pose is known to promote balance and help you focus your attention on the present moment. To practice this pose, follow these steps:

1. Stand and put your feet together, ensuring that your feet press on the ground evenly. Lift yourself up through the crown of your head.

2. You can then lift the thighs and lengthen up through the 4 sides of your waist. In doing so, elongate the spine; and try to breathe easy.

2. Chair or Utkatasana

1. Begin by standing in a mountain pose, and then raise your arms.

2. Now sit back assuming you are sitting on a chair. Shift weight towards the heels, and then lengthen through your torso.

The heating standing pose is designed to strengthen the legs, upper back, and the shoulders.

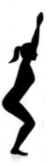

3. Downward Facing Dog or Adho Mukha Svanasana

This pose is designed to open up your shoulders, stretch the hamstrings, and lengthen the spine. It also creates a calming effect as your head is positioned below the heart.

1. Get on all fours, and then walk your hands about one palm length in front of you.

2. Tuck your toes and lift the hips up in order to lengthen your spine. In case you aren't flexible enough, maintain your knees bent in order to bring your entire weight back onto the legs.

3. Now press into the hands, and firm the outer arms. You should reach the upper thighs back towards the wall that is behind you.

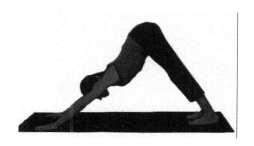

4. Modified Downward Facing Dog

This pose has similar benefits as the initial pose. It incorporates opening of your shoulders, stretching the hamstrings and creating length in the spine. You achieve this without forcing your entire weight on the upper body.

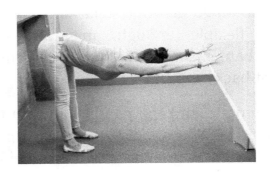

1. Put your hands onto the back of a chair or on a wall or surface with your palms shoulder-distance apart.

2. Step back in order to align the hand under the hips, to create a right angle with your body. Your spine should be parallel to the floor.

3. Now lift through the thighs then firm your outer arms as you lengthen through the crown of the head.

5. Corpse or Savasana

This easy pose is intended to relax your entire body.

1. Lay with your face facing up, separate the legs, and allow your feet to be apart.

2. Position your arms along the sides, and allow the palms to face up

3. Finally close your eyes and try to relax.

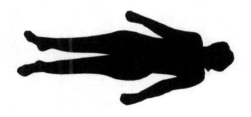

6. Bound Angle or Baddha Konasana

This pose is designed to stretch your groins and inner thighs. The forward bend in this pose creates a cool and calming effect.

1. Sit on the floor, with knees bent but opened wide to resemble a book. Connect the soles of the feet as you sit upright.

2. Position your fingertips onto the ground directly behind you. Now lengthen up though the spine. Alternatively, you can hold onto the ankles and hinge forward at the hips in case your inner thighs feel tight.

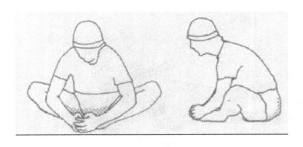

7. Bridge or Setu Bandha Sarvangasana

The bridge pose is helpful in opening your chest and to stretch the neck and spine.

The pose can also help you reduce anxiety, calm the mind and boost digestion.

1. Begin at a lying position with your knees bent, arms at sides and the feet flat on the floor. Keep the feet parallel and hip-width apart. You should stack the heels under the knees.

2. Now roll the upper arms open in order to expand your chest. Through your outer upper arms, ground and root down into the heels. Continue this way until you reach the knees forward to lift the hips from the ground.

3. Shake your shoulders under the chest and then interlace the fingers. In case you find your shoulders tight, try holding onto the side of the yoga mat. This should help you create more space.

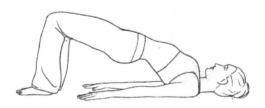

8. Tree or Vrksasana

This pose is useful for improving focus and balance. It helps strengthen the arches of your feet alongside the outer hips.

1. Begin in a mountain pose and then bend one knee. Bring the foot into your upper inner thigh using one of your hands.

2. Alternatively, you can try to bring your feet to the shin below your knee, or instead use a nearby wall for the balance.

3. Then press into the foot you are standing on and lengthen up through your head's crown.

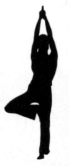

9. Triangle or Trikonasana

The triangle pose is designed to boost your balance, exercise your inner thighs and hamstrings and to allow your body to expand. However, the pose may at the beginning appear to be tough in case you aren't flexible enough.

1. Stand with both of your feet wide apart and then turn left toes in slightly to rotate the right thigh open. Continue until you get the right toes point directly to the side.

2. Ground through the feet and then pull the thighs up; while you keep the legs straight.

3. Spread your arms wide at shoulder height and then roll your front thigh open and now hinge at the front of the hips.

4. Try to lengthen the spine to the direction of the front foot. Release the bottom palm to your front ankle with a yoga block positioned outside your front

ankle. Alternatively, you can just seat on a

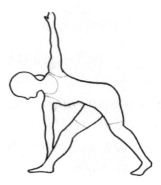

chair.

10. Warrior II or Virabhadrasana II

Warrior pose is meant to calm and relieve a troubled mind, boost your stamina and can strengthen the legs and ankles.

1. Stand with your feet wide, about 3 ½ -4 feet apart.

2. Now turn your left foot in gently, and turn the right foot out 90 degrees to the side.

3. With the arch of your back foot, line up the front heel and then bend the front

knee 90-degree. Use the second toe to track the knee in order to protect your knee joint.

4. Stretch through the straight back leg and ground down into the back foot. Try reaching your arms out to shoulder height, with the shoulder blades positioned down and the palms wide. Then gaze over the front fingers.

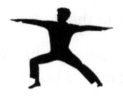

11. Upward-facing Dog or Urdhva Mukha Svanasana

This pose is sometimes considered an intermediate pose as it's a deep back bend that demands for lots of strength.

1. Start from a plank pose, where your feet are hip-width apart, and the arms wide apart then exhale.

2. Slowly, lower your body down using your arms until the elbows form a 90-degree angle.

3. Tilt the body forward using your toes and then roll over the toes in order for the top of your feet to be flat on the floor.

4. Inhale and then straighten the elbow in such a way that the thighs, knees, and torso are lifted from the floor.

5. Ensure that it's only the hands and feet touching the ground. Also look forward, somehow past the tip of your nose.

6. After a few seconds, exit the pose and exhale.

In case you want to easily master the pose, press firmly down using your feet, and continue to draw the chest through your arms. As you pull the shoulders down the back, try to lift from the center of the

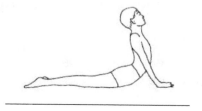

heart.

12. Warrior One (Virabhadrasana 1)

1. Start from a downward-facing dog pose and then step the right foot forward between the hands.

2. Now turn the left heel in and raise up both the arms and torso as you inhale. Ensure that the heel of your front foot is in line with the back of the back foot's arch.

3. Keep the front of the knee just directly over your ankle. Also face both the hips forward, draw the tailbone down as you pull your ribs in.

4. Make sure that the hip's back is facing forward not outward, with the back of the feet being around 45 degrees as opposed to 90.

5. Repeat the warrior 1 pose on the other side of the body.

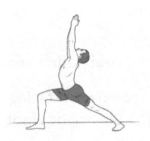

13. Forward Fold (Uttanasana)

The pose is designed to open the back of your legs, and to facilitate the spine to decompress. The pose is also useful in allowing fresh blood flow from the heart into your head.

1. Get into a mountain pose then hinge from your hips on an exhale and then fold

over forward. Try to maintain the spine very straight as you can.

2. Allow the head to hang heavy, and then relax your jaw. You should keep the feet hip-width apart or try to make the feet touch if comfortable.

3. Be aware that keeping the spine straight is more efficient compared to straight legs. Try to bend the knees in order to maintain a straight spine. The chest should touch the thighs. Don't lock the knees but rather try to keep them soft.

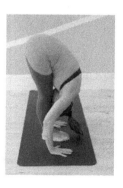

14. Pigeon Pose or Eka pada rajakapotasana

The quad stretch pose helps open the shoulder and the chest. Follow these steps:

1. In a push-up pose, place the palms under the shoulders.

2. Put the left knee onto the ground near the shoulders as the left heel is positioned by your right hip.

3. Now press the hands to the ground and then sit back, having your chest lifted. Alternatively, you can try lowering the chest near the ground for a better stretch. Repeat the pose on the other side.

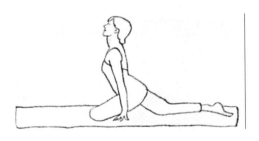

15. Child's Pose or Balasana

The pose is known to help you relax and breathe into your back. It also relieves neck and back pains as it stretches the thighs, ankles and hips.

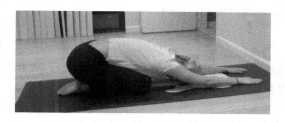

1. Sit upright on your heels and then roll your torso forward.

2. Bring the forehead to rest on the ground just in front of you

3. Now lower the chest to the knees as close as possible, while you extend the arms forward then hold the pose as you breathe into the torso.

4. Now exhale and finally release to get deeper into your fold.

16. Seated Twist or Ardha matsyendrasana

The seated twist is a powerful stretch that you can try out after long durations of sitting in your office. It helps work out the back, hips, and shoulders.

1. Start by sitting on the ground or carpet with extended legs

2. Now close the right foot over the outside of the left thigh and then bend the left knee.

3. Ensure that the right knee faces the ceiling and keep the right hand on the ground behind you. This helps to stabilize your body.

4. Position the left elbow to the outside of the right knee. Then twist to the right as far as possible, as you move from your abdomen.

5. Ensure that both sides of the butt are on the ground. Repeat the pose on both sides.

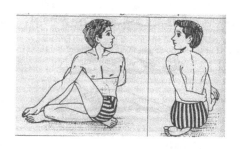

17. Crow Pose or Bakasana

Crow pose is effective at strengthening the abs, arms and wrists. It is quite a challenging pose but with practice, you will be able to pull it off.

1. Start on a downward facing dog pose and then walk the feet forward in order for the knees to touch the arms.

2. Bend the elbows quite carefully as you lift the heels from the ground. Position the knees against the outside of your upper arms.

3. Ensure that you maintain the legs pressed against the arms and the abs engaged. You can also leave the toes on

the floor and instead lift them off and hover. However, ensure that you keep tucked tight; and place the heels very close to the butt.

4. Once ready, push your upper arms against your shins and then draw the inner groins very deep into your pelvis to help

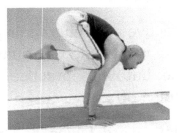

you perform the lift.

18. Plank

This pose is useful in strengthening the core, as it promotes your stability and strengthens the abdominals.

1. Start from the downward facing dog pose and then shift forward in order for

the shoulders to be stacked over your wrists.

2. Now reach the heels back and in the same time, lengthen the crown of your head forward.

3. Ground down into your hands, and pull up through your arms. Spread the collar-bones from your sternum and lift the body to stabilize the pose.

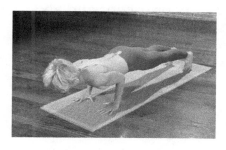

19. Chaturanga Dandasana

1. Begin from a plank pose and then shift forward gently.

2. Bend your elbows around 90-degrees as you place the arms parallel to the ground. Ensure that you support yourself through the palms and spread your collarbones wide.

3. Lift the shoulders from the floor and continue to pull the front ribs into the spine.

4. Lift the upper thighs to the direction of the ceiling and try to reach the tailbone located towards the heels, and then gaze forward.

5. This pose is useful as a part of sun salutation, and helps stabilize and strengthen your triceps and abdominals.

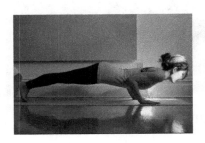

20. Half Moon or Ardha Chandrasana

This pose is effective in strengthening the outer hips and legs. It helps stretch the inner thighs and hamstring, and improves your concentration.

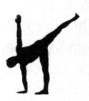

1. Begin this pose from a triangle pose then bend the front knee, as you track it using the second toe.

2. Now step up the back foot in and then walk your bottom hand about 12 inches in front of you.

3. Line up your thumb using the pinky toe as you shift your entire weight into the front foot. Lift the back foot from the floor.

4. Reach to the back leg quite strongly to the direction of the wall behind you as you raise up the top arm.

5. Try to rotate the chest to the ceiling in order to challenge your balance, and then gaze up at your top hand.

As you do the above yoga poses, you will notice an improvement in different facets of your life. This is especially because when doing yoga, you engage different parts of the body. These parts form part of the body's energy centers, famously referred to as chakras. Let's take a brief look on chakras just to help you understand what they are and probably how they relate to different body parts.

CHAPTER 18: DIFFERENT STYLES OF YOGA

Fundamentally, all yoga types and styles strive to deliver the same outcome, the unification of mind, body, spirit and soul. They may vary on their philosophy. Some popular styles of Yoga are:

Hatha Yoga. This kind of yoga style works effectively by focusing on strength building exercises for both mind and physique. It has its root in Hinduism. It incorporates postures, disciplines, gestures breathing and meditation and purification procedures. Hatha yoga is pre-dominantly and popular practiced in West. It is stress relieving practice. Hatha yoga depicts, fire and water, male and female, hot and cold and positive and negative. Its main objective is balancing our mind. Its main focus in on physical movements, breathing and mindfulness and thus, Hatha Yoga brings health benefits. It is a generic term used for physical postures in all kinds of Yoga. It is gentle and slow paced and is introductory step of yoga poses. It leaves the body, loose, relaxed and calm.

Power Yoga (Astanga Vinyasa Yoga). It is popular as modern day version of classical Indian Yoga. It is named after the eight limbs of yoga as described in Yoga Sutras of Patanjali. However, Power Yoga is a generic term for any rigorous yoga style derived from Ashtanga Vinyasa Yoga. It is often referred as 'Gym Yoga'. Power Yoga is a western spin to Ashtanga Vinyasa as it is a series of disciplined and challenging poses styled to boost energy flow and heat. It involves rigorous workout that enhances flexibility and strength. Bryan Kest and Beryl Birch pioneered the introduction of Indian Ashtanga Vinyasa Yoga, with a western touch to it.

Anusara Yoga. Anusara Yoga was pioneered by John Friend, an American Yogi, in 1997. It is a newcomer in the world of ancient Yoga. It is popularized as health oriented Western Approach to Yoga. Anurasa refers to "following through heart; following with nature and 'flowing with grace'. Its practice is classified into three crucial parts, popular as three A's, namely, Alignment, Action and Attitude. It is based on embodying the intrinsic goodness by incorporating physical yoga practices to experience grace, inner goodness and cleansing of soul.

Bikram Yoga (Hot Yoga). Bikram Yoga was popularized by Bikram Choudhary (Founder) by incorporating traditional Hatha Yoga Techniques. This form of yoga is practiced in a heated room, with humidity. It has a series of 26 yoga postures with two breathing exercises. Increased room temperature has a positive impact on the physical performance of the body. Popular benefits of Bikram Yoga are improved posture, increased flexibility, enhanced strength, increase in metabolism and weight loss. It is an excellent detox program as Bikram Yoga flushes the toxins and impurities through sweat from our body. The yoga cleans out the arteries and the veins.

Viniyoga. It is an integrated form of yoga comprising of pranayama, asana, meditation and chanting. It is widely practiced because of its adaptable nature and benefits people of any age. It can be practiced no matter the illnesses, injuries and physical limitations, which you possess. It is characterized by tremendous focus on alignment and consistent number of breaths. It is popular as conventional stretching exercises and eliminates chronic, low-back pain. This ancient Sanskrit term refers to adaptation, appropriate application and differentiation. Vinoyoga stabilizes the sacrum, strengthens the back muscles and balances our spine. It was pioneered by T Krishnamacharya and he passed his legacy to his son T.K.V Desikachar. It works on the principle of proprioceptive neuromuscular facilitation (PNF).

Iyengar Yoga. Iyengar Yoga was developed by B.K.S Iyengar and is a popular form of Hatha Yoga. The main target of Iyengar yoga is to treat disease, ailments and disorders. Iyengar yoga is beneficial for immuno-deficiency, chronic back pain, insomnia, depression, high blood pressure and menopause. This form of Yoga incorporates 200 classical yoga postures and poses and variations of 14 different types of Pranayama. It is different from other styles of Yoga as it incorporates the use of certain props, blocks and belts. It has its roots in the Eight Limbs of Yoga. It is a form of physical therapy, as it works effectively on injured areas.

Raja Yoga. This form of yoga is based to master and quiet the mind's infatuations and hence, is concerned with the mind. It makes the human body fit for meditation, by promoting celibacy, carefully integrated action and abstinence from intoxicants. It prepares the body by depriving it from obsessions and addictions. It is based on Yoga Sutras of Patanjali and hence, this classical Yoga and contains steps such as meditation, contemplation and eventual enlightenment or awakening (moksha). The sole objective of Raja Yoga is to control mental modification and thought-process. It follows the eight limbs of Ashtanga Yoga.

CHAPTER 19: LEARNING ABOUT THE BENEFITS OF YOGA MUDRAS

The mudras are taught in the lesser known and independent branch of yoga that is known as the Yoga Tatva Mudra Vigyan. Mudra is a Sanskrit word that means gesture or attitude. In yoga, mudras are performed in combination with breathing exercises in order to boost the flow of prana and stimulate all parts of the body that are involved in breathing. As you perform the poses, you are slowly creating a subtle connection with your instincts that affect your unconscious reflexes.

There are numerous mudras that range from rare to contemporary. The importance and use of these mudras are taught in Hatha Yoga Pradipika and Gheranda Samhita. The other mudras are tackled and followed in different yoga practices. There are certain mudras that people do naturally without realizing it, such as the simple gesture of touching your hands to your fingers. This kind of gesture brings a subtle change in your attitude and perception. It has some sort of power that can affect and heal your body.

The yoga mudras have a direct relationship with the five elements of the human body. This concept is further explained in Ayurveda. According to Ayurveda, when you suffer from a disease, it means that there is an imbalance in the body that can either be due to the lack or excess of the five elements.

The characteristics of these five elements can be found in your fingers, which make your fingers important electrical circuits. You will use the mudras in order to adjust the flow of energy that has a significant effect in the balance of water earth, air, fire and ether in order to imbibe healing.

Are you ready to learn more about the deeper details of the mudras? Here are some more mudras that you can try and practice with. Before you begin, make sure that you are in a comfortable position. You can either sit on a chair or get into certain yoga poses, such as cross legged, lotus or Vajrasana.

1. Chin mudra

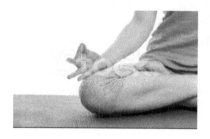

Hold the thumb and your forefinger in a light manner, while the rest of the fingers remain extended and straight. You can place the hands on top of your thighs, with the palms facing up, and wait until you have established your breathing. You don't have to exert any pressure in any fingers. Relax and focus on your breathing. Observe how the process and flow of your breathing affect you.

2. Chinmaya Mudra

Form a ring with your thumb and forefinger, while you let the three remaining fingers curl in your palm. Place your hands on your thighs, with palms facing up. Take deep ujjai breaths, but make sure that you remain comfortable all throughout the process. You will need to focus on your breathing and its effects.

3. Adi Mudra

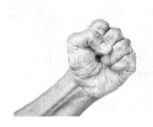

Place your thumb at the base of your small finger, while the rest of the fingers are curled over the thumb, creating a light fist. Like in the first two, put your hands on your thighs, with palms facing up and you will breathe and observe the effects.

4. Brahma Mudra

Place both hands in the position that you have done in Adi Mudra. Put the knuckles of your hands together and place them in the navel area as you keep on breathing and observing its flow.

In order to clearly observe the effects, it is recommended to take at least 12 breaths. Be mindful as to where your breath is flowing and how it affects your mind and body.

In-depth Look into the Yoga Mudras

There are basically two kinds of mudras in yoga. The first one involves the touching of the tips of different fingers with the thumb. The second one is pressing the first phalangeal joint with the thumb. The effects that you will feel depend on which fingers are touching or being pressed. This is due to the fact that the body is composed of different special points that are being targeted by acupressure and acupuncture in order to heal.

Here are the 8 basic hand gestures that are used in yoga and meditation. Some of these mudras have already been discussed in the previous chapter. The following contains more in-depth information about what are these mudras for.

The first two mudras affect the air, the first of the five elements of your body. The air is responsible for your mental health, creativity and intellect. This is associated with Anahata or the fourth chakra.

1. Gyan Mudra

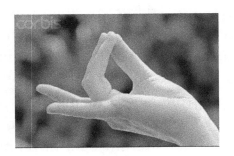

This mudra affects one's wisdom. This is also called Vaayu Vardhak Mudra; Vaayu means air and Cardhak means to enhance. This is done by touching the tips of the

154

index finger with the thumb. In professional yoga, practitioners perform this in order to meditate and disassociate oneself from the material world.

This helps in increasing the element of air in the body. It prompts your creative thinking, enthusiasm and eagerness. When done properly and often, the simple gesture can help in improving your memory and in boosting the cognitive process of thinking. This is also said to alleviate depression, drowsiness and mental retardation. You can practice this mudra anytime and anywhere you are.

2. Vaayu Mudra

It soothes your emotions and makes you feel calm. This is also called Vaayu Shaamak Mudra; Vaayu means air and Shaamak means to suppress. Put the tip of your index finger at the base of your thumb; thumb upon this finger and carefully press it.

This mudra decreases the air element in your body, which in effect, soothes your spirit and calms your mind. It works by pacifying your nervous system and any kinds of hormonal imbalance. This is a recommended activity for people who are hyperactive and aggressive and those who have difficulty in keeping their focus.

The next mudras affect the second element of the human body, which is ether or space. This is subtle and is mostly considered inactive. This is responsible for your collective consciousness and it allows you to resonate with the cosmos. This is mainly associated with Visudda or the fifth chakra.

3. Aakash Mudra

This gives you a feeling of lightness. The term means Aakash or space and Vardhak or to enhance. To perform this, you only need to gently touch the tips of the middle finger with the thumb. The gesture boosts the space element in your body. It eases away your negative thoughts and worries.

It also helps you deal with anger, sadness and fear. It has a detoxifying effect and is ideal for people who often suffer from congestion problems in the tummy, ear, sinus and chest.

For best results, it is recommended to perform this mudra from 2 to 6 in the morning or in the afternoon. If you have an agile body, do not do this for more than 30 minutes each day.

4. Shunya Mudra

This has a healing effect for pains. This is also called Aakash Shaamak Mudra; Aakash means space and Shaamak means to suppress. To perform this, simply touch the tip of your middle finger at the base of your thumb and thumb upon this finger by carefully pressing it.

The mudra decreases the space element in your body. It helps in relieving ear-related pains, such as minor aches, tinnitus, impaired hearing, travel sickness and nausea. It prevents the feeling of numbness in your chest and head. This is recommended for people who have a pronounced Vata constitution. You can do this anytime, but if you are performing this mudra to get rid of ear aches, numbness and vertigo, stop it when you feel that the pain has subsided.

The next mudras are targeted to the Earth element of the human body that is responsible for the physical construction, such as the bones and tissues. This element also governs your nose. The other mudras address the fire element that controls the body's glands, metabolism, growth and temperature. The chakra that is associated with the earth element is the first kind, which is Muladhara. For the fire element, it is the third chakra, which is the Manipura.

5. Prithvi Mudra

This affects one's strength. It is also called Prithvi Vardhak Mudra; Prithvi means earth and Vardhak means to enhance, and Agni Shaamak Mudra; Agni means fire and

Shaamak means to suppress. To do this, simply touch the tips of your ring finger to your thumb.

The action decreases the fire element in your body while boosting the earth element. It allows you to heal, build muscles and encourage growth of new tissue. It helps in boosting your energy and is effective for those who are suffering from dry skin and brittle nails, hair and bones. It promotes endurance and vitality.

This also works by regulating your body temperature and metabolic process. This is recommended to those who are skinny and people who often experience ulcers, fever and inflammation.

6. Surya Mudra

This goes by other names, such as Prithvi Shaamak Mudra; Prithvi means earth and Shaamak means to suppress, and Agni Vardhak Mudra; Agni means fire and Vardhak means to enhance. This is done by placing the tip of the ring finger at the base of the thumb. You will thumb upon that finger by gently pressing it.

It works by decreasing the earth element while increasing the fire element in your system. This is recommended when you are shivering due to low temperature and colds. This is beneficial to those who want to lose weight. It aids in digestion and helps you feel better if you have constipation, suffer from lack of appetite and suppressed thyroid activity. This can be done any time during the day, but do not exceed 30 minutes for each session because it can cause your body to overheat.

Water is the body's fifth and final element. It makes up more than 70 percent of the human body. It has an influence on your skin, tongue, taste, tissues and joints. It corresponds to the second chakra, the energy chakra that is called Swadhisthana.

7. Varun Mudra

This is also called Jal Vardhak Mudra; Jal mean war and Vardhak means to enhance. To perform the action, gently touch the tips of the little finger with your thumb.

This works by increasing the water element in your body. This has a moisturizing effect and is recommended for those who are suffering from general dehydration, cramps and hormonal deficiency.

This helps in relieving joint pains, arthritis and improves the condition of those who have lost the sensation of taste and experience limited body secretions. This works wonders for people with dry hair, eyes and skin, those who are suffering from digestive health problems and eczema. This is safe for everybody except for people who have problems with water retention.

8. Jal Shaamak Mudra

This action, which is intended for stability, means Jal for water and Shaamak means to suppress. Simply put the tip of your little finger to the base of the thumb and thumb upon that finger by gently pressing it.

It works by decreasing the water element in the body. This is recommended for people who have problems with water retention or edema, hyperacidity, too much glandular secretion, watery eyes, sweaty palms, runny nose and too much salivation.

CHAPTER 20: HOW TO UNLOCK YOGA'S SECRET POWER

I am going to take you through some step-by-step yoga poses, or Asanas. So much of what is fundamental to yoga has to do with how you breathe, and how you connect with your breath.

So, I will ask for your indulgence for just a few more minutes while I talk about tapping into the power in your breath.

Let's start with a little background and explanation.

Breathing is as fundamental to yoga as it is to life. We can survive for weeks without food or water, but only a few minutes without breath.

Breathing affects cellular function and brain performance, fuels the burning of oxygen and glucose, which in turn is what sends energy to muscles so they can contract, to glands so they can secrete, and to the brain so it can process information. It is also one of the ways the body gets rid of toxins and waste.

Shallow Versus Deep

The quality of our breath is inextricably linked to the health of both body and mind. The more of our lives we spend shallow breathing, the less healthy we are going to be overall.

Every breath is a gift, according to Eoin Finn, yoga instructor and founder of the Blissology Yoga System. Finn tells the story of how ancient yoga masters thought of our lifetime of breaths as a type of bank account: every deep, relaxing breath is a deposit; and every shallow breath a withdrawal. Based on that analogy, I think many of us would be in overdraft!

The average adult takes over 21,000 breaths every day, and most of those are shallow or low-quality breaths that don't use our full lung capacity.

Think back to the last time you were angry. What was your breathing like? For most of us, being angry or upset brings breathing that is very fast and very shallow.

Now, recall a time when you were feeling calm and relaxed. Can you see how your breathing was different? In a contented state our breath is much more mellow, measured, and yes, relaxed. That's what I want you to aim for.

Pranayama: The Art of Breathing

Yogic breathing, called pranayama, is a powerful tool for human healing. The word pranayama comes from two Sanskrit words: prana = life force, and yama= control/self-control/restraint. Pranayama, therefore, is the controlled regulation of breath.

Through a series of pranayama breath patterns, yoga helps your parasympathetic nervous system activate its 'rest and digest' state (as discussed in Chapter One).

Practicing pranayama teaches you that controlling your breathing can help you control your body, quiet your mind, and reduce stress.

There are three phases of every natural breath:

Inhale: contraction of respiratory muscles

Exhale: passive or relaxation phase, lasts roughly twice as long as inhalation

Pause: the pause after you exhale happens naturally, until an instinct deep within your body triggers the impulse to breathe in – inhaling – again.

Typically, yoga breathing is in and out through your nose, because that is where the air is warmed, moistened and filtered. Think of each inhale as bringing in new life, each exhale as releasing tension, anger, fear and negativity.

Five Pranayama Techniques

There are several different types of pranayama which involve deep breathing, quiet breathing, fast breathing, and more. The five most popular are highlighted here.

Dirga Pranayama

Dirga Pranayama is the three-part breath, a deep and full breathing approach that helps you unlearn the shallow, mouth-breathing that contributes to tension in the body and anxiety in the mind.

The three parts refer to the three distinct areas of your torso into which you will actively draw breath: your low belly, lower rib cage, and upper chest.

The first few times you practice dirga pranayama, it is helpful to rest your hands on each area into which you are breathing to help you isolate each position.

Place your hands on your low belly, the area just under your belly button. Start your first inhale, breathing to expand only into your low belly. Hold this for a count of three.

Move your hands to the sides of your lower ribcage and bring in a little more air so that you can feel your lower ribcage expand, and hold this for a count of three.

Next lift your hands to rest on your upper chest, and bring in the last bit of air and feel the expansion of your upper chest. Hold this for a count of three.

Start to exhale, controlling the rate of your exhale so that you can count to six before your breath is fully emptied from your lungs.

Repeat this process several times, working your way up to a 12-count exhale.

Ujjayi Pranayama

Ujjayi breath is the basic form of breath used in many Ashtanga and Vinyasa classes. It is balanced, both energized and relaxed, and is one of the only pranayama techniques practiced at the same time as the physical postures (Asanas).

The key to ujjayi breath is that you breathe in and out through your nose, making the sound of an ocean wave at the back of your throat without taking in more air. It is a subtle shift in the quality of your breath and takes some practice.

Kapalabhati Pranayama

You'll find this type of pranayama at the end of a Bikram Yoga class.

It starts with a full inhale. Then, with the help of a series of about 15 pulsing abdominal contractions, a forceful exhale empties all the air from your lungs.

After the next full inhale, repeat this forceful exhale between 15 and 30 times, quickly, without taking in another conscious inhale. You will actively contract your abdominals with each pulsing exhale.

After you're finished, return to a few natural breath cycles, before repeating the process for a second round.

Nadhi sodahana pranayama

Also called 'alternative nostril breathing', nadhi sodahana pranayama helps generate equal breath through each nostril while building lung expansion capacity.

To start, clench all the fingers of your right hand into a fist, except your thumb. Press your thumb to your right nostril to close the airflow.

Deeply inhale through the left nostril, and hold your breath.

Change to your left hand, and left nostril, and follow the above steps on the left side.

Repeat the process 15 to 20 times.

Sithali pranayama

This is a cooling breath that can quickly bring your body temperature down.

Start by curling your tongue into a lengthwise tube.

Inhale through this tube, and then close your mouth to the count of 5 or 10.

Breathe out slowly through your nose.

Repeat up to 15 times, and as often as you need to feel comfortably cool.

Tips or Things to Avoid

If you have a cold, asthma, lung problems or heart disease, check with your doctor before you start breath control exercises.

Avoid pranayama when the air is too hot, or too cold.

As often as possible, practice in fresh air, outdoors or with a window open. Avoid polluted or smoky areas, including incense.

Stay relaxed during your pranayama exercises and avoid straining.

Wear loose, comfortable clothing.

CHAPTER 21: THE FUNDAMENTALS OF

PRATHYAHARA

This fifth limb of Yoga advances into the next level of nature. The last four limbs have been fairly structural and tangible in action and understanding. This fifth limb marks the genesis of something more abstract, yet more integral to our existence. Prathyahara is often compared to a turtle in its shell. In this analogy, the shell is the mind and the head and limbs that stick out of it are the senses that are out in the world. When practicing Prathyahara, one retracts all the limbs and head back into the shell to cease input form the outer world.

Why would one need to do this?

The reason is that the mind is an organ of habit. The constant input of various frequencies — sight, sound, and so on, assaults the mind constantly. That is more so today than it was when Yoga was first developed. Today we have all kinds of bells and whistles notifying us of something on our phone, tablet, or computer. We have all kinds of content competing for our attention on the radio, the TV, and the phone. We have unlimited incoming sensations that trigger our minds in so many ways, and they all become a habit. It is the habit of sensory input.

Life in this universe is made up of a simple relationship, the internal and the external. To take advantage of the peace and to develop the path to enlightenment, one needs to master oneself within the context of the universe. The assault of external stimuli prevents us from getting to know our self – one half of the equation.

When one creates the habit of sensory input, it is characterized by the inability to put down the TV remote, log off from YouTube, place your device on silence, or just completely unplug. The current generation of woke individuals calls this the Internet Sabbath. It is a day where they just totally unplug from any external sensory input or data. The first time one does that, the sudden input silence can be overwhelming. It is so because the habit of input needs to be fed or it feels like the cessation of any other bad habit – no different from quitting smoking or getting sober.

Just like junk food, 'junk' habits are inputs that this limb of Yoga is designed to overcome. It has several practices that can be whittled down into three elements. If you recall, Yoga is about matching tangible actions with intangible effects. In this case, the tangible action could be the cessation of certain habits, but the intangible could be the cessation of certain habitual thoughts and perceptions. In the same way, this limb's three elements are categorized into the withdrawal from bad food habits, bad thought patterns, and sub-optimal associative patterns.

Look at it this way: When the body's immune system is strong, the assault of pathogens and parasites in the environment around us are easily overcome. What happens when that immune system is diminished? If that is the case, then even the mildest exposure to pathogens and bacteria will render the body ill. In the same way, if your mind's immune system — its framework and values are diminished, then the slightest exposure to what is ill-conceived will affect the mind, and subsequently the peace that we are in search of.

The objective of his limb is to then achieve objectives in parallel. On one track, it is to abolish the negative input, and at the same time to be in search of positive input. This is where a person's religion can sometimes come into play. Yoga is not a religious endeavor. It is a framework to build the mind and the search for truth and enlightenment.

When you withdraw into the mind, your external exposure is minimized and you are allowed to alter the negative input. At the same time, you are now able to silence the resonating mind that has been placed in a vibration of the negative thoughts.

Look at it this way. If you are in a state of fear while you are at the movies watching a horror flick, until you get out of that theater, or the scene ends, you are not going to be able to begin the process of recovery or normalization. The moment you get out of the theater, the process of liquidating that fear begins. Even though it takes a few minutes, it will eventually get to the point that you are renewed. Stopping the external stimuli is the first move of healing. You can't heal while you are still subjected to the problem.

The same goes for food, thought, and action. In the case of food, your body cannot begin the rejuvenation process until you stop eating what you are habitually consuming. This is the reason, fasting is one of the main actions of the practitioner. Fasting is not just about weight loss, it is also about the health of one's mind. More so, in fact.

When a person fasts, they remove the toxins of the food that they habitually consume, and they reset the habit of

176

eating in the mind. In people who are obese, the problem, when it is not medically or genetically caused, is more psychological. Fasting stops the mind from seeing food the way it did and allows the mind to heal. This healing process will take some time and can be discomforting, especially when it concerns the cessation of food.

The other cessation is about values and practices. These are the actions that we take daily. When we reflect on the values we have and we find them to be in contravention of peace and harmony, what keeps us from rejecting that value? The answer is the habit that we form. To be able to get out from under that burden, we have to retract our senses from the environment that is promoting them.

One method to alter behavior, actions, and practices, is to go on retreat for a week. Change the scenery you are constantly faced with and you will find the impetus to act in a certain way or behave in a certain manner is reduced. That is because the habitual nature of these actions and thoughts is not triggered when you leave the visual cues that evoke a certain characteristic. Think of it this way, when you go to your high school reunion, do you or your friends act the same way you did when you were 18? Even though you are 43 now? You most likely would, because the sight of all the same people triggers you to act the way you did back then.

Retracting your senses from the status quo allows you to heal and take on new habits. This is the lesson of the Prathyahara.

Chapter 22: Yoga Tips For Beginners

To start practicing yoga, you really do not have to be flexible. As a matter of fact, yoga will help you become flexible. Since there are a lot of various yoga styles which range from gentle to vigorous, you may search for yoga instructor and style that will best suit your needs, class schedule, current physical condition, limitations and abilities.

Be sure that your instructor is aware of any health issues and your level of fitness. Do not force any poses or movements. Mastery of yoga poses will come with regular practice. Wear stretchable or lightly loose clothing that are comfortable. Expect to take off your shoes during a yoga session.

At the end of a yoga session, you must feel calm and invigorated and not in physical discomfort. Try attending yoga classes for twice a week or even more. A single yoga session typically lasts for about 60 minutes.

Following are some tips for yoga beginners:

Select a particular yoga type

This step involves doing a little research on your part. A lot of yoga classes are available out there, and you will be most likely to be disappointed if you pick a certain yoga type that does not suit your state of physical fitness and personality.

Take a couple of minutes to read the overview of yoga as provided on the first chapter of this book. For majority of yoga starters, vinyasa or hatha yoga class will be the most suitable, depending on whether you would like to go for a fast or slow-paced class. Keep in mind that these are just basic yoga classes and you can always go for something more advanced or fancier later.

Look for a yoga class

Try looking for yoga classes available in your locality. You may look at online resources, local alternative newspapers as well as wellness and fitness magazines for listings.

Go for a yoga studio that is convenient to your work or home so that it would be easy for you to get into class. Be sure to begin with a basic level yoga class. A lot of fitness centers and gyms also offer yoga sessions – this is a great place to get started if you are already a gym member. Finding a competent yoga instructor will help you to stick with your yoga classes.

Know what to bring during yoga classes

During the first day of your yoga class, you will not have to bring a lot of stuff except for yourself and some breathable, comfortable clothing. Majority of yoga studious have yoga mats available for rental.

Know what to expect

In a usual yoga class, the participants put their yoga mats in a loose grid facing the front of the room. This is usually identifiable by the instructor's mat or a small altar. It is strongly advised not to line up your yoga mat precisely with one next to it since you and your co-yogi will require some space in some yoga spaces. The participants usually sit in a cross-legged position.

The yoga instructor may commence the class by leading the class in reciting the syllable "om" thrice. Depending on the instructor, there could be some short meditation or some breathing exercises at the beginning of the session.

This is usually followed by warm-up yoga poses, then more vigorous poses. Next would be stretches and on to the final relaxation. If you need some rest at any time, take a child's pose.

Oftentimes, the instructor will roam around to every participant during the final relaxation and provide them with a little massage. Majority of yoga instructors end the session with another set of "oms".

The Do's and Don'ts during a Yoga Class

Do's:

Familiarize yourself with some of starter's yoga poses before taking your first yoga session

Ask the yoga instructor for help if you need it

Inform your yoga instructor that it's going to be your first yoga session

Review yoga etiquette so that you will feel very comfortable in a very unfamiliar situation

Come back in a couple of days for your next yoga session

Don'ts:

Wear socks or shoes during yoga sessions

Drink water during the session, although have some before and after the class

Have a good meal right before a yoga session. Try to eat light a couple of hours before the session begins

CHAPTER 23: YOGA POSES FOR WEIGHT LOSS

Downward-facing Dog

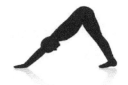

Along with the upward-facing dog, this asana is one of the most famous and frequently done pose no matter what type of yoga you are into. This asana will stretch your hamstrings, calves, hands, and shoulders and will strengthen your arms and legs.

Begin with planking down your body on the mat, face-down. Then, put your palms on your sides as if you're about to do push-ups. Put a foot of distance between your left and right foot. In your next exhalation, straighten your arms and lift your buttocks upwards towards the ceiling. Your hands and feet must be parallel to each other.

Your legs should be straightened out. Proceed to moving your chest closer towards your knees so that the crown of your head will be near, but not touching, the floor. You have option to either keep your back straight or bending it from the base of your spine.

Try to hold this pose for 1 to 3 minutes with your gaze concentrated beyond your feet.

Setu Bandh (Bridge Pose)

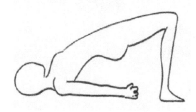

First, you have to lie flat on your back on the floor. Then, bend your knees so that the soles of your feet are resting on the floor. During your next exhalation, press your arms and feet into the floor, pushing your tailbone and lifting your buttocks off the floor.

Clench your hands and straighten out your arms in order to stay on the tops of your shoulders. Next, you should lift your buttocks until your thighs are parallel to the floor.

Lift your chin slightly away from your chest and firm your shoulder blades against your back. Hold this position for 1 minute.

Dhanurasana

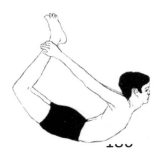

Lie down on the floor facedown. Then, put your hands besides your chest and then lift your legs and thighs upwards. Meanwhile, try catching the legs you lifted upwards with your hands. Hold this position for 30 seconds before releasing.

Shalbasana

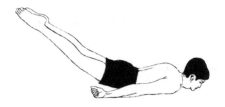

Lie on the floor facedown, keeping your hands rested below your thighs. Your forehead and chin must be resting against the floor. Next, lift your legs up, keeping them straightened out. Remember not to bend your knees. Hold this position for 1 minute.

Chakki Chalan (Grinding Pose)

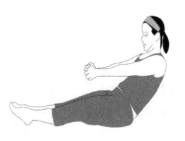

This asana is an effective exercise for reducing belly fat. Start with sitting down on the floor in a comfortable position and spreading your legs straight in front of you. Now, your right and left leg should be touching each other and your knees should not be bent. Then, recline your body backwards a little bit and join your hands in front you, clasping the fingers together. Afterwards, move your joint hands in a circular motion over your legs. Do this movement twenty times first in clockwise position and then in counter-clockwise.

Nauka Chalan (Boat Pose)

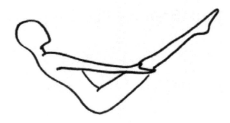

The boat pose will target and strengthen your back and abdominal muscles. This certain asana will help you reduce the fat around your waist.

First thing you need to do is to sit down comfortably on the floor. Then straighten your legs in front of you while keeping your hands by your side. Next, recline your torso backwards as you simultaneously raise your legs until both your feet are a foot higher compared to your head. The ankles of your feet should be touching each other. Make sure that your weight is balanced on your buttocks and not on the lower part of your spine.

Your arms must be extended straight past your knees and must be parallel to the floor with your palms facing inward. Hold this pose for 30 seconds if you can.

Now, move both your hands forward and backward while moving your torso in the same manner. Do these 20 times and release afterwards.

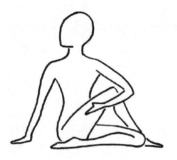

Ardha Matsyendrasana

Sit down on the floor with your legs straightened out in front of you. Then, bend your knees and place your feet on the floor. Put your left food under your right leg with the outside part of your leg touching the floor. At this point, your right foot must be over the left leg and place it near your left hip. Then, place your right hand against the floor behind your right buttock. Meanwhile, your left arm must be on your right thigh or somewhere near your right knee. Make sure that your right knee is pointed directly upwards.

Turn your head to the right. Hold this position for 30 seconds before releasing.

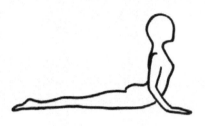

Bhujangasana (Cobra Pose)

As the name suggests, the form you must take for this pose resembles a serpent. The first thing that you have to do is lie face down on the mat with your forehead touching the ground. Next, put your palms under your shoulders and stretch your legs until both your feet presses down into the floor. As you inhale, gradually press your hands against the floor to stretch your arms, sending your upper torso or chest upwards. Hold this pose for 30 seconds.

Padahastasana

Start by standing up straight. Your feet must be touching each other. Next, as you exhale, bend downwards as far as you can and touch your feet with your fingers. Slip your fingers under your feet as you make sure that your arms are stretched. Hold this position as long as you can before slowly rising upwards and going back to the first position.

Trikonasana

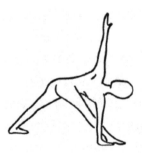

Stand up straight and keep your feet wide apart. Now, turn your right foot to a 90-degree angle while turning your left foot to a 15-degree angle. Then, you have to bend your body to the right and downward from your hips. Remember that your waist must be kept straight. Lift your left hand up in the air while put your right hand on the ground. Keep both arms in a straight line.

Paschimottanasana

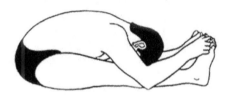

This pose is ideal for reducing extra belly fat and it demands effort on the part of your hands, arms, and spine.

Sit down on the floor and straighten both of your legs in front of you. Stretch your arms and torso forward as far as you can. Try to touch your left toes. Remember that you must not bend your left knee as you try to reach your toes. Hold this position for 1 minute.

Tadasana (Mountain Pose)

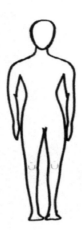

The mountain pose is usually used in the beginning or ending of a yoga sequence and can also be utilized as a transitional asana. It's one of the easiest postures that anybody can add to his yoga program.

Start with standing on both feet. Keep your feet together. You can also opt to put a little bit of distance between them if you have trouble balancing with your feet touching together. Then, extend your arms along the sides of your body and tilt your head up slightly.

Ustrasana

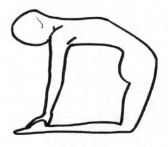

This pose requires the backward stretching of your spine. It demands a kind of flexibility in order to maneuver this move. First, you have to kneel on the mat with your thighs and feet touching each other. Proceed to placing your palms on your hips. The thumbs of your hands must be touching your lower spine. Next, curve your torso backwards and then place your palms on your feet. Make sure that your palms on your soles. At the same time, stretch your chest forward.

With your palms on your feet, stretch your head back as far as you possibly can. Hold this pose for 30 seconds.

Utkatasana (Chair Pose)

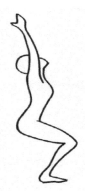

Begin with the Tadasana (mountain) pose. Then, stretch both your hands up in the air. Afterwards, bend your knees downwards, ensuring that your thighs are kept parallel compared to the floor. Try to imagine sitting on a chair, that's what this pose will look like.

196

Hold this position for 30 seconds to a minute before releasing.

Phalakasana (High Plank)

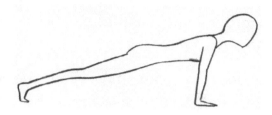

Begin with lying face down on the ground. Now, lift your arms up as if you're doing push-ups, bringing your whole body upwards. You must keep your arms straightened out, with your palms pressing against the floor and the toes of your feet ensuring your balance.

Hold this position for 30 seconds.

Lunge

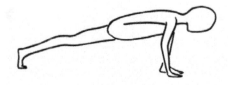

Sit straight with your legs touching each other. Now, step forward using your right leg and bending it in the process. Move your right leg forward as far as you can. Your left leg must be kept straightened behind you.

Place both of your palms on the mat directly under your shoulders. Hold this position for 30 seconds to 1 minute.

CONCLUSION

After reading this a book I guess that you have had a fun with it, I hope that you have found what you are seeking for, is to make your body and mind feel very fresh and comfortable especially your back body. Hoping you happy journey with your happy life and good health.